Borders and Healers

EDITED BY
TRACY J. LUEDKE

AND

HARRY G. WEST

Borders and Healers

Brokering Therapeutic Resources in Southeast Africa

INDIANA UNIVERSITY PRESS
Bloomington and Indianapolis

This book is a publication of

Indiana University Press
601 North Morton Street
Bloomington, IN 47404-3797 USA

http://iupress.indiana.edu

Telephone orders   800-842-6796
Fax orders   812-855-7931
Orders by e-mail   iuporder@indiana.edu

© 2006 by Indiana University Press

The paper used in this publication meets the minimum requirements of American National Standard for Information Sciences—Permanence of Paper for Printed Library Materials, ANSI Z39.48-1984.

Manufactured in the United States of America

Library of Congress Cataloging-in-Publication Data

Borders and healers : brokering therapeutic resources in southeast Africa / edited by Tracy J. Luedke and Harry G. West.
      p.   cm.
   Includes bibliographical references and index.
   ISBN 0-253-34663-0 (cloth : alk. paper) — ISBN 0-253-21805-5 (pbk. : alk. paper)
   1. Traditional medicine—Africa, Southern. 2. Healing—Africa, Southern. 3. Therapeutics—Africa, Southern. 4. Body, Human—Social aspects—Africa, Southern. 5. Africa, Southern—Social life and customs. I. Luedke, Tracy J. II. West, Harry G.
   GT497.A356B67 2005
   398'.353—dc22

                                                                          2005015437

1 2 3 4 5   11 10 09 08 07 06

Contents

Acknowledgments

This volume emerges from a dialogue sustained among its contributors over a period of two years. The group first convened as a panel at the 101st annual meetings of the American Anthropological Association in New Orleans in November 2002. Participants in the panel included volume contributors Christopher Colvin, Stacey Langwick, Tracy Luedke, James Pfeiffer, David Simmons, Rijk van Dijk, and Harry West. Karen Flint, Robert Marlin, and Sheryl McCurdy also presented papers, and commentary was provided by Richard Werbner and Megan Vaughan. Following this, a working group was convened in Philadelphia, with support provided by the African Studies Center at the University of Pennsylvania, where papers were discussed in greater detail. Ellen Foley and Tonya Taylor joined the working group, as did Steven Feierman, who served as discussant. Special thanks go to Tonya for facilitating the group's assembly in Philadelphia as well as to Tonya, Christy Schuetze, and Ellen Foley for hosting members of the group in their homes.

Borders and Healers

Introduction
Healing Divides: Therapeutic Border Work in Southeast Africa

Harry G. West and Tracy J. Luedke

In Xipamanine's marketplace, in among the fruits and vegetables, the live chickens, freshly butchered sides of beef, and dried fish, the "wholesalers" of Johnny Walker Red Label and Orange Fanta, the vendors of bootlegged audio- and videocassettes, the hawkers of handmade reed mats and faux-Naugahyde loveseats, and the photo-takers and letter-writers, there are healers at work. In this place of densest circulation in the most populous neighborhood in the capital city of Mozambique (Maputo), the business of healing thrives. Some healers can be found sitting on the ground behind bamboo partitions, performing divination to diagnose the cause of their clients' misfortunes. Others display on wooden tables before them animal skins, bits of dried roots and tree bark, bottles containing variously colored powers, and cloth packets whose contents remain a mystery to the browser. Still others engage in conversation with individuals or with groups assembled around them—sometimes in conspiratorial tones and sometimes in the voices of preachers.

Xipamanine's healers all seem to come from elsewhere, whether another neighborhood, a distant province in central or northern Mozambique, or a foreign country such as Swaziland, South Africa, Botswana, Congo, or Nigeria (see also Meneses n.d., 17). Some dress as cosmopolitan travelers—the men sporting flashy polyester shirts and sunglasses and the women wearing makeup and decked out in jewelry. Others dress as "peasants in the big city"—the men wearing darkly colored sport coats over simple T-shirts and the women wrapped in *capulanas* and headscarves. Some display their "credentials" (including "training certificates" and government licenses), prescribe "dosages" of carefully labeled substances, and perform "medical procedures" such as "vaccination." Others rely for their reputations on word of mouth and specialize in engaging unseen forces such as disgruntled ancestral spirits, witches, or Satan. As indicated by the frequency with which they are consulted, many of these healers inspire the confidence of their clients. Judging by the gossip among city residents, many also inspire fear.

While many of the healers in Xipamanine have traveled great distances to set up their practices in Mozambique's largest market, their journeys are emblematic of a broader phenomenon among healers in Mozambique and throughout the region of southeast Africa today. In the rural town of Mueda in northern Mozambique, where one of us (West) has conducted ethnographic field research since 1993, the most respected "local" healers include several who were either born across the border in Tanzania or who claim to have learned their vocation there. In Angonia (in central Mozambique), where the other of us (Luedke) has worked since 1998, the most popular healers are prophets possessed by biblical spirits; they appeared only after the recently ended war in Mozambique, having acquired their healing abilities during their time as refugees in Malawi. Healers, it would seem, are often judged more powerful on the other side of the border—which is where many of them, not surprisingly, wind up (Last 1992, 39; Prince and Geissler 2001, 455; Rekdal 1999, 459; Whyte 1982, 2061; Whyte 1988, 226; see also Pigg 1996, 194n7).

The healers of Xipamanine, Mueda, and Angonia cross not only literal boundaries but figurative ones as well. If boundaries can be said to exist between the rural and the urban, the local and the global, the official and the unofficial, and the traditional and the modern; between ethnic groups, languages, and religious communities; and between religion and science, the material and immaterial worlds, and healing and harming, then healers, it would seem, cross boundaries constantly. In Angonia, for example, despite official ambivalence toward them, individual healers claim a state mandate for their practices by affiliating themselves with a healers' association, based in Maputo, that links them across geographical and metaphorical divides with the nation's urban center of power and with global development networks. In Mueda, "traditional healers" incorporate into their healing repertoires practices they identify as "scientific," such as keeping patient registers and charting rates of success. Further, many of Mueda's most respected healers consult the Koran and depend for guidance upon *majini* spirits (genies), notwithstanding the fact that their clients nearly all identify themselves as Christians. So fundamental to the profile of the healer are transgressions of boundaries that one might conclude that the power of healing is in some profound way bound up with the act of crossing borders (Rekdal 1999; Whyte and van der Geest 1988, 7).

Such was the idea that we posed to our colleagues whose essays appear in this volume. The topic seemed to us quite urgent, for we and our colleagues—each of whom works on issues related to health and healing in southeast Africa—had all borne witness, in recent years, to a series of interrelated crises which have negatively impacted the health and well-being of most of the region's residents.[1] Civil wars in Mozambique and Angola were the legacy not only of violent struggles for independence against the Portuguese but also of attempts by white settler regimes in Rhodesia and South Africa to undermine majority rule in the region in the late 1970s and early 1980s. While the vast majority of African residents of South Africa and Namibia experienced dire poverty under apartheid rule—and were generally denied access to quality state-funded health care—the governments of neighboring "frontline states" were forced to divert resources away from social services such as health care and toward military defense. Periodic drought and environmental degradation—exacerbated by massive flows of refugees—further contributed to the state of emergency throughout the region. With the end of the Cold War came the end of Eastern bloc support for socialist regimes in southeast Africa. By 1994, most nations in the region—including South Africa—boasted multiparty political regimes; most had also assented to IMF-sponsored structural adjustment programs that mandated significant cuts in social services. Notwithstanding enhanced regional security and economic growth, standards of living have since fallen for most people, who often find the goods available on the "free market" beyond their means. Corruption and/or popular suspicions of graft have characterized these neoliberal states, which have all but abandoned the public project of development. Simultaneously, greater regional stability and intensified commerce have eliminated preexisting barriers to the spread of the HIV virus. In short, the interrelated catastrophes the region has suffered have been felt acutely in the realm of health and healing. Besides bringing about the collapse, in many countries, of health care networks constructed by post-independence states (Andersson and Marks 1989; Cliff 1991; Cliff and Noormahomed 1988; Cliff and Noormahomed 1993; Feierman 1985; Pfeiffer 2002; van der Geest 1997, 903), these crises have placed the institutions of kinship and community, through which people might seek relief, under enormous strain. Under these desperate circumstances, residents of the region have been compelled to piece together disparate therapeutic resources in an attempt to meet their health needs. In so doing, they have looked, where possible, to the far side of the boundaries with which they have been confronted. We therefore urged our colleagues to consider not only how the various healers with whom they have worked transgress boundaries but also how, in so doing, these healers generate and/or deploy the power that animates their healing practices.

Our preliminary conversations provided persuasive evidence of the extensive circulation and concomitant border-crossing of the people and spirits, objects and substances, practices and techniques, discourses, ideas, and memories associated with healing in southeast Africa. As Megan Vaughan (who contributed to these early conversations) pointed out, however, such forms of circulation are nothing new to the region, nor, indeed, were our collective accounts of them anything new to the regional literature on health and healing (cf. Rekdal 1999, 463). Evidence abounds from as far back as the historical record reaches of the movement across geographical and social borders of healers and their patients and of the materials and ideas associated with healing (van Binsbergen 1995; Whyte, van der Geest, and Hardon 2002, 6–9). In the early nineteenth-century, for example, London Missionary Society director John Campbell observed among the Twsana a propensity to—as John and Jean Comaroff have paraphrased him—"[search] out cures [among neighboring African people] to enhance their own therapeutic repertoire" (Comaroff and Comaroff 1997, 338; see also Rekdal 1999, 473 in reference to the Iraqw of Tanzania, and Whyte 1982, 262 in reference to the Nyole of Uganda).[2] In *Witchcraft, Oracles and Magic among the Azande*—the first substantial ethnography of an African people ever written—Evans-Pritchard recounted that the Azande imported *benge* (the poison substance administered to chickens within the context of oracular divination, a fundament of Zande cosmology) from across the border in the Congo (Evans-Pritchard 1937/1976, 156). In the mid-1930s, Audrey Richards provided accounts of witch finders in the region whose modus operandi was to "[cross] the border from some neighboring territory with all the kudos attached to the foreign and the strange," "to appear, as if from nowhere, flourish for a time, and then disappear" (Richards 1935/1970, 201; see also Marwick 1950; Probst 1999; Willis 1968). As Vaughan has observed, healing practices and techniques circulated even between Africans and Europeans in their early encounters; she writes: "African healing systems showed themselves to be remarkably resilient and adaptive. Far from being destroyed by the joint assault of colonialism and biomedicine, they tended rather to absorb and internalize, to 'indigenize', those elements of biomedical practice which seemed most effective and most impressive—the most obvious being the injection" (Vaughan 1991, 24;[3] see also White 2000, 99–101). By the same token, Europeans have long adapted—"indigenized"—elements of African healing as well; John and Jean Comaroff write that "whites who lived along the perimeters of Rolong, Tlhaping, and Tlharo communities [in the late 1960s] . . . set great store by *setswana* herbal remedies, some of which they purchased directly from healers; the rest were bought from tiny, unkempt shops, usually situated in those gray areas of small towns where 'European' trade gave way to commerce of legally indeterminate color" (Comaroff and Comaroff 1997, 364).[4]

If, however, charting the circulation of personae, objects, and ideas associated with healing in Africa is nothing new, neither was it our principal objective in convening our colleagues. In conceiving this volume, we hoped to explore the relationship between such forms of circulation and the force that healers derive from them—to examine how border-crossings of various kinds empower healers and make the work of healing possible. Nonetheless, Vaughan's critique gave us cause for reflection. If the stuff of healing has long been in circulation—if circulation and border-crossing are, in fact, the norm rather than the exception in this region—then the continuing existence of such borders is as noteworthy as contemporary crossings of them. We began to suspect that the power of healing was bound up in important ways with both of these phenomena: border-crossing *and* the persistence of borders.

It was this question that animated continuing conversations in which we reflected on the fact that for decades now, the term "traditional medicine" (or "traditional healing") has been subjected to critique by the very people who study the phenomena it delineates (Feierman 1985, 110–112; van der Geest 1997, 904). The cause for our shared discontent with the term, of course, is that it conjures up the boundaries that we so regularly see healers cross. "Traditional medicine" suggests discreet and enduring practices associated with social groups demarcated by common residence, descent, language, social status, and/or religious belief and distinguishable from other discreet and enduring practices associated with other such groups—a notion belied by the broad regional exchange of healers, and their substances and practices, that we have witnessed. What is more, the term suggests that these practices are mutually exclusive with "official," "modern," or "scientific" forms of healing, despite the fact that we regularly see these boundaries crossed as well. All of us are well versed in the argument that "tradition is dynamic"—a mantra that is, by now, a tired cliché among anthropologists and other social scientists. The scare quotes that inevitably adorn the term are widely understood to convey recognition of tradition's dynamism. We were equally familiar with more sophisticated arguments about the way in which tradition and modernity historically emerge in tandem as a dichotomous pair, dependent upon one another for their existence (e.g. Pigg 1996). What vexed us was that the more we problematized the term "traditional medicine" (and each of us had done so at one time or another in print or in debate around a conference table), the more resilient it proved itself to be. Attempts to craft a new language with which to speak about these issues generally ended, we all knew, in demands from a confused audience to decode our new terms and eventually to confess that it is, after all, "traditional medicine" that we are talking about.

The persistence of "traditional medicine" in the face of relentless critique makes it impossible simply to dismiss the term. Instead, we realized, it is important to distinguish between "traditional medicine" as a failed analytical category and "traditional medicine" as a resilient, polyvalent "folk category" that is deployed by a multiplicity of folk, including social scientists, representatives of international health organizations and development institutions, biomedical practitioners, and state officials as well as, revealingly, healers and their patients. Here, we follow James Ferguson, who suggests the need to conceive of analytical tropes—he uses the example of "modernization"—not as external to the social field to which they have been historically applied but instead as objects of study in their own right. He writes: "On the one hand, the narrative of modernization was always bad social science; it was (and is) a myth . . . resting on fundamental misperceptions about the modern history of urban Africa. But, on the other hand, the myth of modernization (no less than any other myth) gives form to an understanding of the world, providing a set of categories and premises that continue to shape people's experiences and interpretations of their lives." Ferguson's approach emphasizes "the continuing relevance of older theories to events that they fail to account for—the way social-scientific theories and cognate folk understandings of the past haunt the present."[5] In seeking to understand how "traditional medicine" haunts the southeast African present, we thus asked ourselves in what contexts and to what ends diverse categories of people in the region continue to use the term.

By approaching "traditional medicine" in this way, we came to realize that the use of the term by and about healers reveals an investment in the (re)production of the boundaries it implies. We concluded that healers, their clients, and analysts interested in delineating and defining their activities, all (re)construct the boundaries around "traditional medicine" even as they challenge and cross them.[6] This realization gave rise to the fundamental argument animating this volume: insofar as the power of healing is bound up with crossing borders, it is also, necessarily, bound up with the construction and maintenance of these borders. In the end, we have come to view border-crossing and border (re)production not as contradictory activities but rather as mutually dependent—indeed, mutually constitutive—acts.

Healers, we suggest, invariably position themselves as mediators between domains to whose (re)production they actively contribute. They derive force, to be sure, from ferrying back and forth between these domains, but their power as healers depends also upon the inability of their clients, and their competitors, to make the journeys—literal and/or figurative—that they do. Successful healers "broker" (Rasmussen 1998, 167) access to therapeutic resources otherwise unavailable or inaccessible to their clients—resources over which they claim privileged, or exclusive, access. As brokers (Somé calls such figures "gatekeepers," 1998, 75; see also Sharp 1993, 208), healers both facilitate and deny people access to specific therapeutic resources. At some moments they import therapeutic substances, practices, or ideas from one domain to another; whether the resources they tout are officially sanctioned or not, they seek clients by "advertising" their wares (Cocks and Dold 2000, 1506). At other moments, by contrast, they seal off these resources so as to prevent the diffusion of their own authority, "closing off flows" (Geschiere and Meyer 1999, 2), be they global or local. Healers, therefore, exploit borders in varied ways. Their boundary work entails moving and crossing—as well as policing—boundaries (cf. Gieryn 1983).

The notion of boundaries is clearly spatial in nature, even when extended to discussions of figurative or social boundaries. Indeed, we suggest that literal and figurative borders are intertwined and conflated with one another in many complex ways and should therefore be addressed in tandem.[7] The anthropological literature on globalization is relevant here, as it theorizes the dialectic between the dissolution of old boundaries and erecting of new ones—boundaries that are often simultaneously physical and conceptual. Appadurai (1996) has famously suggested that the contemporary world is characterized by "global cultural flows"—"scapes" of various sorts that undermine previous notions of bounded social or cultural entities. Geschiere and Meyer point out that "global flows" are often paired with "cultural closure," as the destabilizing effects of global flows drive people to reinforce old, and create new, social boundaries (1999, 2). The circulation and boundary-crossing associated with modernity afford enticing opportunities but also often threaten bodily and social well-being.[8] In the more specific context of African healing, literal and figurative boundaries are frequently intertwined, as bounded spaces are often necessary for the construction of a healing community.[9] Given the salience and danger of boundaries and boundary-crossing for Africans, we suggest that healers, through their special engagement with these boundaries in their physical and conceptual travels, exploit sources of power that few others dare to.

In emphasizing healers' agency here, we follow Feierman and Janzen's mandate to "describe African medicine in the active voice" (1992, 12). This is not to suggest that healers' agency is always apparent. While the contributors to this volume provide evidence of strategic innovation and political maneuvering on the part of healers, they also offer provocative examples of healers who assert that they practice by means of a force that transcends them, whether God (see also Mahlke 1995), ancestral spirits (see also Abdool Karim, Ziqubu-Page, and Arendse 1994; Whyte 1997, 61), divining tools (cf. van Binsbergen 1995; Werbner 1989), or medicinal substances (see also Probst 1999, 117; van der Geest 1997, 909). Many healers profess to serve merely as mediums by which these higher forces are manifest. For many, in fact, the power to heal first alighted upon them in the form of debilitating illness (see also Janzen 1992; Rasmussen 2001a; Whyte 1997, 61, 113);[10] they came to be healers through suffering, they assert, and not through intentional acts (see also Meneses n.d., 10; Stoller 1989, 122). While in some instances a discourse of passivity may be deployed strategically, it cannot be dismissed in toto as disingenuous. However, even as becoming a healer, like falling ill, is something that happens to one, the patient-turned-healer may enthusiastically embrace the role and actively pursue its realization. This, then, is another of the fundamental divides that healers both transcend and reify: the divide between suffering patient and soothing healer.

In any case, because the value of healers' brokerage depends in part upon limited access to the resources they dispense, healers are deeply invested in the maintenance of the very borders they cross. Given that ordinary Africans seek to circumvent therapeutic gatekeepers—both official and unofficial—by acquiring medicinal substances and using them to self-medicate and treat family and friends (Cocks and Dold 2000), successful healers must act not only as cross-border travelers but also as border guards, regulating and restricting the flow of the resources in which they traffic as well as the flow of potential competitors and the clients for whom they compete. Indeed, in many ways healers *constitute* the borders they work, bringing them into existence through their demarcating and patrolling acts.[11]

The idea of the healer as border-crosser and border guard—indeed, as border embodied—underlies and animates what is novel in our approach to, and original in our conclusions about, healing in contemporary southeast Africa. Where the existing literature has provided valuable evidence of the circulation of healers and their techniques and tools, it has tended to conceptualize this circulation in terms of movement from one bounded domain to another. In other words, it has taken for granted the existence of boundaries and the distinct domains they circumscribe, including "traditional medicine" or biomedicine, science or religion, spirit possession or Christianity or Islam, and things African or European or Asian. For some, these bounded domains have been understood to exist side by side, in the same social space, as options from which citizens of a "medically plural" society might choose (Brodwin 1996; Good 1987; Ingstad 1989; Janzen 1978; Janzen 1985; Obbo 1996, 199; Swantz 1989).[12] For others, movement across these boundaries has been understood to erode divides or reconfigure domains. Scholars have for some time theorized this in terms of "syncretism"—the blending of once-distinct systems that yields new, mixed systems (Greenwood 1992).[13] More recently, many have conceived of circulation as a phenomenon contributing to the "hybridization" of systems.[14] Such approaches, however, have all been predicated upon the assumption that distinctive systems exist (or at least existed at some point in time); in fact, they take such distinct systems as their analytical point of departure (e.g. Prins 1992; cf. Cocks and Dold 2000).[15]

Given the historical depth and intensity of circulation in the region, it makes little sense to us, however, to take distinctive systems and the borders between them as our starting point. Such an approach treats as aberrations the realities that we—and residents of the region—encounter.[16] We begin our analysis instead with a landscape comprising therapeutic resources of diverse provenance—resources that are widely (albeit unevenly) distributed.[17] We view this landscape not by means of a map of compartmentalized domains telling us where we might expect to find certain resources but instead through the acts and experiences of healers, patients, and other social actors who encounter these resources as they exist on the social landscape and (re)arrange them into new constellations. Rather than taking for granted the existence of boundaries, we seek to discover how bounded entities are produced and reproduced in the practice of healing.

The contributors to this volume achieve this in a variety of ways. Some follow life histories—or career histories—of particular healers or document component events of these biographies (See Langwick, West, this volume). Others detail the historical emergence of particular healing cults, associations, or institutions (See Luedke, Simmons, this volume). Still others provide accounts of the ways in which healers have brokered—that is, facilitated and/or obstructed—the movements of specific therapeutic resources, whether they be objects or memories, substances or techniques (See Murchison, Colvin, this volume).[18] The approaches the contributors to the volume take allow them to move beyond the truism that "tradition is dynamic" and explore instead the contemporary dynamics—the means and ends—of a variety of healing practices in southeast Africa today.

The authors examine a wide variety of actors associated with healing in this region, including sorcerers and spirit mediums, herbalists and injectionists, church leaders and representatives of healing associations and medical institutions. These various healers craft for themselves disparate "styles," to use James Ferguson's terminology (1999).[19] Whereas some embrace or otherwise seek to accommodate local categories such as "traditional doctor," "prophet," "diviner," or "witch finder," many work assiduously to transcend the bounds of locality, of indigeneity, and of tradition (see West, van Dijk, this volume; see also Geschiere 1998, 821; Whyte 1988).[20] Some dispense, draw upon, or mime the resources of "official," "modern," or "biomedical" institutions[21] or position themselves as the purveyors of healing resources associated with Christianity or Islam, while others distinguish themselves from all that is "foreign" to their constituents, drawing power from domains to which exogenous actors have limited access (see also Obbo 1996, 187, 198; Pigg 1996, 170).

8 *Harry G. West and Tracy J. Luedke*

Whereas all healers broker therapeutic resources for their patients, some healers also act as brokers in their relationships with other healers, mediating the ways healers conduct themselves as individuals and as a group in relation to the broader society of which they are a part. In addition to portraying the pursuits and accomplishments of individual healers in relation to their patients, the chapters provide evidence of healers acting on this broader social scale through institutions and organizations, including healers' associations (see also Green 1996; Last and Chavunduka 1986; Waite 2000), churches (see also Comaroff 1985; Devisch 1996; Kiernan 1976a; Kiernan 1976b; MacGaffey 1983), "cults of affliction" or "*ngoma*" (see also Devisch 1993; Honwana 2002; Janzen 1992; Turner 1968; van Dijk, Reis, and Spierenburg 2000a), and organs of the state (see also Green 1996; Last and Chavunduka 1986; Waite 2000). These organizations and their leadership are often implicated in the activities of individual healers, at times facilitating and at times constraining them. They are sites of differentiation among healers where distinctions are drawn between leaders and followers and/or between experienced mentors and neophytes or patients on the way to becoming healers. It is through these organizations that some healers assert themselves as "political entrepreneurs" (Bayart 1993, 207–272),[22] positioning themselves as leaders by regulating practices and cultivating constituencies (see Luedke, this volume). For example, prophetic healers attract patients whose illness management requires induction into their congregations, leaders of healers' associations bring healers together as a social body while at the same time policing and controlling their activities, and these same leaders lobby health ministries and other government agencies in order to secure a place for "traditional medicine" in national policy planning. Healers, then, often act as brokers in two registers, one at the level of the healer-patient dyad, the other at the level of social bodies of healers and patients.

Regardless of strategy or style, whether working with individual patients or as leaders of social bodies, healers' powers depend upon innovation and creativity (Last 1992, 404; Rekdal 1999, 472; Whyte 1988, 226). Although some healers learn about medicinal plants from masters with whom they apprentice, they still must scour the landscape in search of new healing substances or develop new uses for known substances; they often achieve this by traveling and trading substances and knowledge with other healers near and far. Most healers aver that the effectiveness of the medicinal substances their masters and colleagues pass on to them depends upon their own abilities to craft a unique operative relationship with the forces that animate these materials (Davis 2000, 232; Reynolds 1986, 173; van der Geest 1997, 909; cf. Whyte 1997, 28).[23] Healers conceive similarly of spiritual and/or occult forces. Healers who learn about medicinal plants from spirits engage in an ongoing apprenticeship in which the spirits reveal new information as new healing situations arise. Healers may work with the spirits of recently deceased relatives or with the spirits of long-departed ancestors whose public memory they sustain or, sometimes, even reactivate. Healers who work with spirits widely known for their healing prowess demonstrate their ingenuity by cultivating distinctive relationships with them (Lambek 1993, 305–337; Sharp 1993, 115–120). Healers who work with spiritual entities of foreign provenance, such as Christian spirits or saints or coastal Islamic *majini* (Janzen 1989, 240), show their innovativeness in accommodating these lesser-known forces.[24] Other healers display their originality by incorporating into their practices elements drawn from biomedicine or from transregional consumer culture.

For healers, innovation often entails introducing patients to objects, substances, practices, or ideas with which they are unfamiliar and controlling the process whereby patients are familiarized with these entities. Healers who draw on exogenous resources clearly act as brokers of the unfamiliar, but healers embracing a more "traditional" style often also play this role, locating the unfamiliar in dreams, spirit domains, and/or archaic languages and thereby asserting their unique capacities as mediators of the (even to their patients) strange forces contained within these realms. In any case, a healer's innovation must be buttressed with evidence of "competence" (Ferguson 1999, 98). Whereas healers who fail to innovate—who administer resources that are too familiar to their clients—risk a loss of client confidence (people in Mueda say "that one's medicine has grown stale"), healers who journey too far afield in their quest for novel resources may have trouble persuading clients of their grasp over these resources or of the credibility of the resources themselves (Ngubane 1992, 373). Perhaps more important, the unfamiliar forces and resources that healers deploy must not be altogether unrecognizable to clients (see Colvin, this volume). Novel objects, substances, ideas, and techniques applied to healing must resonate in some way with familiar sites and sources of power (Rekdal 1999, 472; Whyte 1982).[25] Resources applied to healing may be familiar to varying degrees, reflecting a range of possible time depths from which elements may be drawn. Repetition and consistency in healers' practices may allow for the construction of a community with a sense of identity or of a following with a sense of security. Reaching farther back, healers may draw elements from recent history, including events, personalities, and objects that have figured in the lives of participants. Healers may reach even farther back in time, drawing elements from a remote past that echoes only faintly across generations but nonetheless resonates with healers and patients in the present (Sharp 1993; Shaw 2002). Healers' innovations may involve deploying something from the past in a new way or inserting a new element into an old method. In responding to these new combinations, people may be seeking access to the foreign and exotic (Prince and Geissler 2001, 455), but they may also be reaching out for something that is somehow familiar. Healers weave together the known and the unknown— mining the unfamiliar within the familiar and vice versa.

The resonating force of historical precedent may be manifest in healing practices in rhythms and melodies, scents and tastes, comforts and ordeals that work on the sensate body but defy the intellect (Brown 1989, 257; Clammer 2002, 46; Friedson 1996; Rasmussen 2001a, 101–130; Roseman 1988; Roseman 1991; Stoller 1996). The semantic load carried by healing objects, substances, techniques, and ideas is sometimes only dimly perceived, whether by healer or by patient (Rasmussen 2001a, 128). While healers sometimes explain to their patients the logics that animate healing practices, often they do not, or cannot (see West, this volume). Patients may be left to discuss and debate the meaning of healing practices among themselves or simply to accept them without explanation (Last 1992; cf. Davis-Roberts 1992, 385). The power of such healing practices and the way they are experienced is as much a product of their mystery as their "sense."

As brokers of such forms of power, healers are often cast—or cast themselves—as knowers of the unknowable. Discussions of "traditional medicine" often assume "knowledge" to be the resource upon which healers' claims of authority and legitimacy rest. The model of "indigenous knowledge" touted by advocates of "traditional medicine" suggests the equation of knowledge with certainty. Many healers, however, "know" medicines, spirits, and diagnostic tools only in the sense that they are acquainted with them; they often assert, in fact, that they do not understand precisely how these things work. Several of the chapters in this volume emphasize that healing knowledge is neither easily possessed nor uncomplicatedly implemented (see Murchison, West, this volume). On the contrary, they suggest that healing knowledge is inherently unstable and difficult to control. Healers do not simply acquire and use knowledge; they are engaged in a constant struggle with it (Whyte 1997, 81–82).[26] Knowledge of this kind, in fact, may be empowering precisely by virtue of its ambiguity and unwieldiness; power, in the understanding of many in the region, adheres as much to the unknowable as to knowledge. In some cases, knowing may in fact be undesirable because of the complex moral and political implications associated with certain kinds of knowledge (Last 1992, 400). In any case, the paradoxical claim of many healers to know the unknowable and the contradictory assertions of others to know and at the same time not to know suggest that familiarity and unfamiliarity are better understood as graduated, mutable, and multifarious states rather than as paired opposites.

Yet as brokers of the unfamiliar, healers nonetheless spawn dichotomous pairs and the borders between them even as they transgress these borders. On the ever-shifting horizon that healing practices construct between the familiar and the unfamiliar linger the social categories of those who know and those who don't (see Fernandez 1982, 68), those with access and those without, and those who can cross over and those who cannot. These categories give rise to and reinforce distinctions between social selves and social others, including patrons and clients (see van Dijk, this volume); the rich and the poor (see Pfeiffer, this volume); the powerful and the weak; the urban and the rural; the formal and the informal (see Simmons, this volume); the modern and the traditional (see Langwick, this volume); one community of believers, kin, or citizens and another; and the righteous and the immoral. Insofar as healers facilitate and/or restrict their clients' access to novel therapeutic resources, they articulate their clients' affinities with and/or differences from others who use these resources.

In focusing on how healers access, reject, adapt, deploy, and control the varied therapeutic resources on the southeast African landscape today and how they produce and/or capture power through these maneuvers, the contributors to this volume simultaneously chart the emergence and transformation of borders *and* the social categories they demarcate. A more pressing mandate for the study of healing in the region could scarcely be imagined. As mentioned above, people living in southeast Africa today daily experience the effects of interrelated crises. So profound are the combined effects of the current economic, political, and social malaise that residents of the region generally experience crisis not as a passing episode but rather as a perpetual state of being. Within the context of this unending state of siege (Taussig 1992, 11–35, following Benjamin 1968, 257, who calls it a "state of emergency"), residents of the region have become adept at exploiting any and every therapeutic resource they encounter. Healers in particular have developed an acute sense of emerging and transforming power relations, seeking whenever and wherever possible to improve their positions vis-à-vis a vast array of social others. Our readings of healers' practices and maneuvers thus contribute to a deepening understanding of the vectors and gradients of power along which social categories and relations are constituted in contemporary southeast Africa.

In Chapter 1, Harry West opens with an account of how the Mozambican state, after years of "socialist modernization" and official repression of "obscurantist" healing beliefs and practices, now celebrates "traditional healers" as a national heritage. The transition, West argues, derives from the collapse of the socialist project after years of South African destabilization, followed by the post-apartheid, post–Cold War ascendance of neoliberalism, which permitted the government to reimagine healers as low-cost local human resources. West suggests, however, that policy reform has failed to produce substantial collaboration between the official health care system and "traditional healers" owing to misconceptions rooted in the indigenous knowledge paradigm that animates such reform. Whereas this paradigm conceives of healers as the bearers of rarefied empirical knowledge that might be harvested, validated, and used by biomedical researchers and practitioners, the "traditional healers" with whom West worked in Mueda district were interested neither in providing data to health researchers nor in preserving their indigenous/traditional purity. Indeed, West argues, the power and local legitimacy of these healers *depended* upon their abilities to transcend the bounds of locality, of indigeneity, and of tradition—to draw upon forces rooted on the other side of the geographical, social, and cosmological borders they (re)produced through their healing practices. According to West, biomedical researchers and practitioners remained wary of Muedan "traditional healers" not only because of their border transgressions but also because the *knowledge* these healers brokered was irreducible to empirical data, drawing instead upon partial visions of a hidden domain of sorcery defined by capricious and ultimately *unknowable* powers.

Like West, Tracy Luedke writes of healers in the charged environment of post-socialist, postwar Mozambique, but she focuses on how they position themselves as authorities and leaders by means of an array of institution-building strategies. Included among the refugees returning from Malawi to Tete Province after the end of the Mozambican civil war were *aneneri* prophet healers who simultaneously provided their clients access to Christianized healing spirits and afforded returnees a means of maintaining linkages across geopolitical borders to a land that had been their home for, in many cases, more than a decade. Although they are a novel cultural form to the region, *aneneri* employed locally understandable power-building strategies and engaged with existing social/political forms. *Aneneri* acted as "mothers" to clients in whom they discovered spirit/host potentialities, giving rise to family hierarchies at whose apex they positioned themselves. Others founded "churches" within which they took titles such as "bishop" and "reverend." Still others occupied positions as "presidents" at various levels in the nascent Mozambican Traditional Medicine Association, often in combination with their standing as "mothers" or "bishops." The "families," "churches," and "bureaucracies" which *aneneri* created and/or inhabited not only challenged but also derived power from their association with the institutions upon which they were modeled. Indeed, the most successful *aneneri* were able to parlay the authority of the state or Christian churches into new forms of *aneneri* power and vice versa. Such entrepreneurial maneuvers blurred the boundaries around official institutions as well as those between institutional and individual power, even as *aneneri* made of themselves stewards of these borderlands.

In Chapter 3, David Simmons continues the focus on healers' associations, examining how the Zimbabwe National Traditional Healers Association (ZINATHA) has mediated between healers and the state by registering and monitoring the work of its members. By Simmons's account, ZINATHA has not only offered training courses to aspiring healers but has also run clinical trials on medicinal substances and packaged them for commercial distribution—in some cases labeled with "modern" names such as "A.C.T.5," "GK 17," or "Profferon" and with "dosage" instructions. As Simmons points out, ZINATHA and its member-healers walk a fine line: seeking through "modern" means to validate their standing as "traditional healers," they risk being condemned as neither modern nor traditional. Indeed, clients look upon ZINATHA's entrepreneurialism—and the novel recombining of elements it entails—with ambivalence. Yet in working the border between modern medicine and traditional healing, ZINATHA healers speak to the predicament of their mostly urban clients, making sense of the possibilities and constraints of modernity by constructing a neotraditional position between "tradition" and "modernity."

The next two chapters further the theme of social bodies as vehicles for therapeutic border work. Both examine African Independent Churches. The first, by James Pfeiffer, also engages with a healers' association (the same Mozambican Traditional Medicine Association discussed by Luedke and West). Pfeiffer offers evidence that within the context of post-socialist structural adjustment and economic liberalization, the commodification of healing—both "traditional" and "modern"—has produced deep anxieties among residents of the central Mozambican town of Chimoio. Pharmaceuticals are sold at exorbitant prices in shops and clinics as well as in/on the (black) market, and "traditional healers"—buoyed by the Mozambican Traditional Medicine Association—extract outrageous fees from clients. In this climate, African Independent Churches and Pentecostal movements have thrived, offering congregants— including, especially, women with limited cash incomes—alternative therapy that is "cost-free" (notwithstanding the sometimes considerable financial obligations of church membership). While partially occupying the niche of "traditional healers," church leaders and prophets have distinguished themselves from these healers—who traffic in forces that can be used to harm as well as to heal— by asserting themselves as agents of a morally unambiguous Holy Spirit. Through demonizing "traditional healers," Pfeiffer tells us, these church leaders and prophets give foundation to church power by (re)drawing the line between good and evil.

Rijk van Dijk writes of two Pentecostal churches in Botswana: the Bible Live Church International and the Christ Citadel International Church. Whereas others have cited the transnational mobility of Pentecostal churches as an example of globalization, van Dijk interests himself in the regionally specific dynamics of the spread of Pentecostalism. It is ironic that the success of these churches in Botswana has been contingent upon shifting state policies designed to "renationalize" professions—ranging from health care to law to education to hairdressing—filled for decades by expatriates from neighboring countries and from Nigeria and Ghana who were recruited to assist Botswana in the building of a modern nation. To the extent that these churches lay the foundation for people subjected to increasing state-sponsored xenophobia in Botswana to craft for themselves a transnational identity, they appeal to labor migrants such as the Ghanaian beauty-salon owners at the center of van Dijk's analysis, who find themselves suffering the affliction of being "stuck in the nation." In other words, these churches not only cross borders, they also allow their members to transcend borders even as they stay put. In this context, van Dijk suggests, church leaders—many of whom are businessmen/women—act as "religious entrepreneurs," not only among expatriate members but also among Batswana. According to van Dijk, Pentecostal churches have, in recent years, become as fashionable among Batswana as the West African hairstyles that Ghanaian church members have brought with them to Botswana for decades, appealing as they do to the transnational cosmopolitan aspirations of local people.

Julian Murchison's chapter, which follows, offers occasion to consider how people respond to health-related anxieties not only through attempts to transcend the local but also through attempts to seal borders and localize healing powers and practices. Murchison's chapter is also the first of three focusing on discursive practices as therapeutic border work. Murchison analyzes stories he collected during the conduct of fieldwork in southern Tanzania about a local woman giving birth to a box labeled "Dawa ya Ukimwi" (AIDs medicine/ cure). In telling and retelling the story, Murchison suggests, Tanzanians (and the spirits said to have provided the cure) asserted agency in the midst of the AIDS pandemic through the elaboration of a hope-filled narrative imaginary in which not only did a cure emerge from within the very body of an ordinary rural Tanzanian woman but it also proved effective only when administered within the district where she resided—a district that tellers of the story associated with "deep tradition." According to these stories, the curing substance resisted biomedical testing, validation, and appropriation, flowing from its container only when in the presence of a patient that *it* diagnosed as afflicted with *ukimwi*. In (re)producing such accounts, Murchison suggests, rural Tanzanians transgressed and sometimes reconfigured boundaries between the traditional and the modern, the foreign and the local, the comprehensible and the incomprehensible, and the curable and the incurable, all the while calling into question the exhausted claims (in the face of the AIDs pandemic) of biomedicine and positing the existence of other forms of power/knowledge directly accessible to (at least some among) them.

Stacey Langwick continues the focus on discourse as therapeutic border work through her examination of the narratives of Dr. Leader Stirling, a Scotsman who first traveled to Tanganyika in 1935 under the auspices of the Universities' Mission to Central Africa (UMCA) but who took Tanzanian citizenship at independence and was later named minister of health. Langwick reminds us that Europeans have long acted as healers on the African landscape and that they too have endeavored to bolster their authority through the (re)production of borders. Through a critical reading of Stirling's published works, Langwick recounts his attempts to give foundation—quite literally—to biomedical claims of superiority over an other of its own invention, namely "traditional medicine." Stirling—like other European missionary doctors of the time—rendered the dichotomy between biomedicine and "traditional medicine" material through the construction of medical facilities designed to separate an African world of untamed natural elements and human superstitions from a European one of scientific order, equipping operating rooms with improved ceilings and observation windows in order to keep infectious agents (including patients' family members) at bay. In his observations on "traditional healing," Stirling further policed the dichotomy between traditional and modern medicine by sometimes validating the efficacy of selected substances used by healers while simultaneously condemning such figures as entirely unscientific. However, even as Stirling patrolled the boundary between these two domains, Langwick tells us, he was often compelled to reluctantly mediate relations between them, allowing—sometimes even encouraging—would-be clients to find echoes of the familiar in his own practices.

Chris Colvin, like Langwick, interests himself in a particular Western discourse about illness and healing and the way in which this discourse has interacted with African understandings and practices. Specifically, Colvin examines how various South Africans have adapted, deployed, and/or rejected "traumatic storytelling" as a therapeutic resource in the post-apartheid era. In Colvin's biography of traumatic storytelling, foreign nongovernmental agencies deemed traumatic storytelling an apt means of addressing South Africa's violent past without forcing awkward, costly, and potentially destabilizing social changes, while the post-apartheid state used traumatic storytelling to manufacture a national narrative of reconciliation between repentant perpetrators and forgiving victims. After the close of the Truth and Reconciliation Commission (TRC), however, traumatic storytelling became an object of social contestation and transformation as it was redeployed and/or spurned by various social groups. At the Cape Town Trauma Centre for Survivors of Violence and Torture, where Colvin conducted fieldwork, group members considered traumatic storytelling a constraint to discussion of continuing everyday problems. In time, the Trauma Centre's support group for torture victims, with whom Colvin also worked, came to focus not on the production of a narrative of reconciliation but rather on efforts to address contemporary social problems stemming from the apartheid past and on the quest for reparations (promised, but not yet delivered, by the TRC). To this end, members of this group, called Khulumani, used traumatic storytelling as a tool toward further ends, presenting evidence in support of their demands for financial compensation in the now-familiar genre of trauma. In doing so, Colvin tells us, group members brokered their own healing as they saw fit, contesting tidy official boundaries between past and present, between the old state and the new, and between the unhealed and the healed, not to mention between well-resourced care providers and underresourced victims.

The volume closes with an afterword by Steven Feierman which situates its contributions within broader discussions of healing in the anthropological and African studies literatures.

Notes

1.   The trends we witnessed were by no means exclusive to southeast Africa. Particular historical circumstances have perhaps rendered the dynamics we describe more visible—and thus more amenable to study—than elsewhere, but colleagues working in other world regions will no doubt recognize these interrelated crises. We hope that they will also find various aspects of our analysis useful as they approach similar issues in the regions they study.

2.   Guyer's (1996) discussion of African "traditions of invention" is relevant here. Guyer suggests that a fundamental characteristic of precolonial equatorial African societies was the fostering of originality, creativity, and difference through societal endorsement of "constant and volatile engagement" with the "boundless frontiers" of known social roles, skills, practices, and ideas (1-2).

3.   By way of example, Vaughan tell us that soon after a Church Missionary Society campaign in 1898 to vaccinate people against smallpox in and around Jilore, an African healer began vaccinating people against the threat of lion attacks (Vaughan 1991, 59; see also Whyte 1997, 26; Whyte, van der Geest, and Hardon 2002, 104-116). Africans also made medicines of a variety of

powerful foreign substances associated with Europeans: when nineteenth-century Tswana men encountered the gunpowder of Wesleyan missionaries, they "perform[ed] an experiment in the mimetic manufacture of European pharmacopoeia. Having observed that whites ingested nothing much raw, they 'cooked' the 'seeds' in the hope of producing a potent distillate. In the upshot, which was very potent indeed, gunpowder came to be known as . . . 'the exploder's medicine'" (Comaroff and Comaroff 1997, 338). Likewise, traditional healers who worked among the communities of black mine workers of 1930s Johannesburg mixed blasting gelatin, "that most potent medicine of the white man," with herbs and used the mixture for therapeutic ends (Lewis in Dauskardt 1991, 89).

4. Work from a number of scholars of South African therapeutic practices suggests that the use of medicinal substances across social, ethnic, and racial boundaries has been standard practice for a long time. Dauskardt (1991) documents the emergence of "herbal pharmacies" in Johannesburg in the 1930s and 1940s. The shops were typically owned by Indian traders and stocked both unprocessed medicinal plants and factory-produced herbal remedies. Cocks and Dold (2000) describe contemporary *muthi* stores in eastern Cape Province which carry herbal and animal-based traditional medicines; commercialized, mass-produced herbal remedies; modern over-the-counter pharmaceuticals; Dutch and Afrikaner folk remedies; and manufactured remedies originating from India, China, and Japan. Du Toit (1998), in his research with elderly residents of Cape Province, found that they indeed drew on an array of therapeutic substances reflecting the healing traditions of both Africans and European settlers. See also Probst (1999, 113).

5. Similarly, Ranger describes how the "traditions" that European colonizers invented for Africans and that Africans invented for themselves (often drawing on the neotraditions European colonizers invented for *them*selves) "distorted the past but became in themselves realities through which a good deal of colonial encounter was expressed" (1983, 212).

6. Bashkow's discussion of boundaries is instructive here. He reminds us that not all boundaries serve as barriers; they are by definition, however, sites where differentiation is actively (re)produced (2004, 450).

7. Bashkow reminds us: "[N]ot all cultural boundaries can be represented in maps. Some of the most important ones must be conceived of as abstract typological distinctions" (2004, 451). A number of studies that address the social phenomena in and around physical and geopolitical boundaries are useful for thinking about the more figurative boundary work of the healers we discuss. For example, in his work on the U.S./Mexico border, Kearney (1991) discusses both the official mediators of the border, the state, and the informal mediators, the "coyotes," who are paid to lead groups of illegal migrants across the border. Kearney points out that El Coyote is "the supremely ambiguous and contradictory trickster" and thus a fitting hero of the liminal borderlands (62). Kearney recalls Turner's concept of liminality, the "betwixt and between" stage in ritual transformation (Turner 1967, 93–111). Flynn (1997) describes life on the Benin-Nigeria border, where residents have laid claim to the borderlands as their own and seek to mediate all

cross-border flows. The Shabe border residents she describes understand the power of their interstitial position and make of it a "deeply placed stable identity" (Flynn 1997, 312–313). These works reveal the border as a conceptual and/or physical space, inhabited by intermediary figures who assist laymen in navigating the promise and danger of the border. They recognize borders as constructed and contested, as sites of creativity and challenge (cf. Hannerz 1997).

8. For example, in her work on Niger, Masquelier has shown that roads are perceived with a great deal of ambivalence by local people, objects of "both fascination and terror" (2002, 831). On the one hand, roads are understood to bring jobs, goods, opportunities, and development; on the other, they bring marginalization and isolation. Drivers obtain amulets and medicines to guard against the "cruel and bloodthirsty spirits" who inhabit the road and threaten travelers. White (1997) suggests that stories about the circulation of heads and other body parts across "political and conceptual boundaries" cause and reveal Africans' anxieties regarding boundary-crossing. Further, and against recent claims of the increasing dissolution of political and economic boundaries, Ferguson reminds us that for Africans especially, recent history has been marked by the entrenching of barriers. Current political and economic realities leave many Africans distanced, both physically and symbolically, from the world community (2002, 559). Thus one's ability or inability to cross literal boundaries often depends on and in turn informs the social boundaries one is able to cross.

9. Devisch describes how the leaders of charismatic healing churches in Kinshasa hold their meetings in spaces physically bounded off from the modern world with palm leaves: when participants arrive at the entrance they must "turn away from the world" (1996, 578). Similarly, Scarnecchia reports that when newcomers arrived at the entrance to Mai Chaza's religious healing community in 1950s Rhodesia, they were met by assistants who registered their names and required them to confess their sins before entry to the compound was permitted (1997, 93).

10. Eliade (1964) referred to this phenomenon as the "wounded healer" (cited in Reis 2000, 62).

11. Some healers occupy roles at once official and unofficial. For example, van der Geest describes government officials and health workers whose trade in medicines on the black market redraws the boundaries between official and unofficial medical realms (1988). In her work on the "middle figures" in colonial medicine in the Congo, including, for example, African midwives, Hunt describes acts and actors who bridged the social boundary between colonizer and colonized (1999).

12. Feierman and Janzen (1992, 4–5) suggest that "the history of healing is a history of multiple traditions, each one with its own distribution in time and space" but that people more readily draw from multiple healing traditions than they do from, say, religious traditions.

13. Shaw and Stewart have addressed the problematic notion of "syncretism," suggesting that this concept is best understood not as accurately descriptive of certain kinds of religious forms but as a discursive tool used by various actors to define similarity and difference (1994, 6). Both syncretism and anti-

syncretism (the shoring up of religious boundaries against synthesizing tendencies) can be used to claim authenticity or charge inauthenticity (7–9). They point out that these claims and charges are often associated with the "innovators" and "entrepreneurs" involved in novel or shifting religious forms (17).

14. Leslie speaks of "cosmopolitan medicine" (1976, 8). See Purcell and Onjoro (2002, 165) for a discussion—with references—of the use of similar terms such as "incorporation," "blending," "fruitful accommodation," "articulation," and "integration." See also Ellen (2002, 243). On the phenomenon of "creolisation" more generally, see Hannerz (1987).

15. Rekdal (1999) attributes this to the colonial-era investment of administrators and structural-functionalist anthropologists alike in the idea of bounded "tribes" whose existence gave foundation to distinct "traditions" that could be juxtaposed with the singular modern world. See Last (1992) for a critique of the idea of traditional medical "systems." Last in fact characterizes Hausa traditional medicine as a thriving "nonsystem."

16. Ellen usefully reminds us that "what is hybrid knowledge for one generation is indigenous in the next" (2002, 243).

17. Similarly, Bashkow points out that the great variance of isoglosses—lines demarcating the currency of *particular linguistic features*—challenges the idea of bounded linguistic domains (2004, 451–452).

18. Several contributors have heeded Whyte, van der Geest, and Hardon's call (2002) to treat medicines as things with social lives by approaching a variety of therapeutic resources—including paradigms such as post-traumatic stress disorder (see Colvin, this volume)—in this way.

19. Ferguson suggests that Africans today chose between "traditional" and "cosmopolitan" styles in many spheres of life. We suggest that healers contribute to the production of an ever-changing constellation of styles.

20. As Ute Luig points out (1999, 137), the very notion of the local is (re)produced and transformed by both types of healers.

21. Simon and Lamla describe Xhosa healers wearing white lab coats and stethoscopes and conspicuously displaying shelves of medical publications as they dispense penicillin (1991, 239).

22. In his discussion of postcolonial African political life, Bayart (1993) suggests that the entrepreneurial accumulation of power takes place at all levels of society and that "this competition is the very stuff of political life" (211). Would-be leaders of various sorts and various scales, including, we would suggest, healers, operate within the same sociopolitical environment and draw on the same set of political tactics (Bayart 1993, 219, 249).

23. See also Bates (1995, 3), who differentiates between gnostic ways of knowing (dependent upon the person of the healer) and epistemic ways of knowing (in which method is emphasized).

24. Boddy reports that spirits of foreign provenance have become standard members of the Zār pantheon and new spirits continue to appear (1989, 275–230, 359). In a number of contexts, diverse local spirits have been transformed into the generalized Christian spirit entities of the Holy Spirit and Satan (Fry 2000; ter Haar and Ellis 1988).

25. As Bashkow, paraphrasing Sapir, suggests, "the foreign itself is incorporated

within the very cultural perspective from which it is seen as external" (2004, 452).

26. Whyte writes: "Divination not only attempts to resolve . . . uncertainty; it also contributes to its maintenance by providing a framework for it. Both uncertainty and its resolution are generated in divination" (1997, 82).

1 Working the Borders to Beneficial Effect: The Not-So-Indigenous Knowledge of Not-So-Traditional Healers in Northern Mozambique

Harry G. West

When I first decided, after several years conducting anthropological research in Mozambique, to focus my attention during a 1999 research stint explicitly on healers, I paid a visit to the Ministry of Health in Maputo before heading north to my field site on the Mueda plateau in Cabo Delgado Province. I was somewhat surprised by what I heard from one ministry official: "Traditional healers are the stewards of a Mozambican medical cornucopia," she told me. Days later, an officer of the Cabo Delgado Provincial Directorate of Health echoed this perspective: "Traditional healers are Mozambique's doctors and Mozambique's medical textbooks," he averred. When I arrived in Mueda, the district director of health added his own endorsement to these views: "Traditional healers know cures for diseases that Western medicine cannot heal," he told me proudly. "They even know cures for diseases that Western medicine has not yet diagnosed."

The views expressed by these officials reflected a dramatic reversal of the official position on "traditional healing" in Mozambique. In the years following Mozambican independence in 1975, the socialist FRELIMO (Frente de Libertação de Moçambique) state had sought to establish a national health system that would provide basic biomedical care to residents of even the remotest villages (Cliff and Walt 1986). The regime cast traditional healers as "obscurantists" whose primitive and superstitious practices undermined the project of "socialist modernization" of the countryside (AMETRAMO 1998; Green, Jurg, and Dgedge 1993, 264; Green, Jurg, and Djedje 1994, 7; Honwana 2002, 169–173). From the late 1970s, however, FRELIMO socialism had met with violent opposition in the form of RENAMO (Resistência Nacional Moçambicana) insurgents backed by the white settler regimes of Rhodesia and South Africa (Finnegan 1992; Hall 1990; Minter 1989; Morgan 1990; Vines 1991).

By the end of the 1980s, the socialist project—including hundreds of rural health clinics—lay in ruins (Cliff and Noormahomed 1987; Cliff and Noormahomed 1988). As FRELIMO moved toward a negotiated peace with RENAMO—

necessitating constitutional reform and the transition to multiparty democracy—the government also came to terms with the International Monetary Fund on a structural adjustment support package (Hanlon 1991). Although it was victorious in the nation's first national elections in 1994, FRELIMO possessed neither the resources nor the will to reconstruct socialist-era health programs in a post–civil war era defined by the end of the Cold War, the end of apartheid, and the global ascendance of neoliberalism. The government instead took cues from international donors and nongovernmental organizations which espoused "democratic decentralization" and the "empowerment of local communities" to solve their own problems and meet their own needs. It was within this political and economic climate that government officials such as those with whom I conversed came to speak of traditional healers not as subversive delinquents but instead as low-cost local human resources.

Even in the early 1980s, the Mozambican government had shown some interest in traditional healing. Paradoxically, while the state expressly prohibited the practice of traditional healing, researchers in the Ministry of Health's Department for the Study of Traditional Medicine (Gabinete de Estudos de Medicina Tradicional, GEMT) gathered data on medicinal plants used by healers throughout the country.[1] In the mid-1980s, the ministry published a four-volume catalogue of Mozambican medicinal plants and their various uses in the practice of traditional healing (Jansen and Mendes 1983–1984). During the heyday of Mozambican socialism, however, a strict boundary was established between *medicinal substances,* which might be of scientific value, and *healers,* whose practices were generally deemed incompatible with scientific medicine.

In 1990, the European Union provided funding for a consultant—American medical anthropologist Edward Green—to advise the Mozambican Ministry of Health on policy formation and legislative reform in relation to traditional healers (Green 1994, 121). Green questioned the GEMT focus on *materia medica*[2] and challenged the GEMT notion that traditional healers were inherently "unscientific." Green counseled it to distinguish not between healers and the potentially valuable substances they used but between magic and the often valuable distinctive forms of local knowledge that traditional healers preserved and deployed in their practices. He argued that researchers and health practitioners alike had long overemphasized the magical components of African notions of health and healing (Green 1999). He wrote: "[I]ndigenous and biomedical etiological models are, in fact, not very different in fundamental and important ways" (12). Seemingly exotic cultural expressions, he argued, worked as symbols (or as metaphors); once decoded, he asserted, these expressions were altogether compatible with biomedical categories and concepts of disease and its treatment (16, 18, 90). For example, African concepts of pollution constituted an "indigenous contagion theory," Green suggested; and the "invisible snake" (which many southern African peoples suggest resides in the body of a healthy person)[3] constituted an "indigenous theory of resistance" to disease (1997, 1999).[4]

Building upon the "traditional medicine" paradigm elaborated by the World

Health Organization from the mid-1970s onward (Bannerman, Burton, and Wen-Chieh 1983; World Health Organization 1978; World Health Organization 1995), Green argued that the "indigenous knowledge" possessed by Mozambican traditional healers made their participation in collaborative research and health care an invaluable national resource. "A society's creativity and genius is embodied in its IKS [Indigenous Knowledge Systems]," Green wrote. "An understanding of health-related indigenous knowledge is . . . essential for health planners and implementers, if plans and programs are to be culturally appropriate and therefore effective" (1994, 21).

To that end, Green proposed that the government adopt the World Health Organization definition of "traditional medical practitioners," that it allow these practitioners to form associations, and that it recognize the members of legally constituted associations (1994, 124–125). In 1991, with Green's assistance, the GEMT "proposed a three-year program to begin public health collaboration between the National Health Service and the indigenous health practitioners of Mozambique" (Green, Jurg, and Djedje 1994, 8). The U.S. Agency for International Development (USAID) subsequently funded field studies undertaken by Green and a team of researchers working in the GEMT to examine existent and potential contributions of traditional healing to the prevention and treatment of sexually transmitted diseases and infant diarrhea (Gaspar and Djedje 1994; Green, Jurg, and Dgedge 1993; Green, Marrato, and Wilsonne 1995).

In 1992, the Mozambican Traditional Medicine Association (Associação da Medicina Tradicional de Moçambique, AMETRAMO) was formed with the approval of the Mozambican state. In subsequent years, state administrators and health officials throughout the country nominally recognized members of the association. However, the collaboration envisioned by Green and other advocates of traditional healers was not forthcoming. When I visited with the president of AMETRAMO for Cabo Delgado Province in 1999, he informed me that he sometimes received visitors—foreign and Mozambican—who asked permission to gather *materia medica* from association members, but he lamented that these visitors abruptly disappeared without sharing the findings of their research or the profits he was certain they garnered. Beyond this, he told me, there was no collaboration between AMETRAMO and the official health care system. When we asked the assistant president of AMETRAMO for Mueda District about forms of cooperation between the association's healers and the district hospital, she bemoaned the fact that while healers sometimes referred clients to the hospital, the hospital never sent patients to healers. Notwithstanding the pronouncements of health officials from Maputo to Pemba to Mueda who now spoke of traditional healers and their knowledge as a national heritage, these officials continued to look upon traditional healing and traditional healers with deep suspicion and/or contempt.

A closer look at the indigenous knowledge paradigm suggests why this should be so. As Arun Agrawal has pointed out, indigenous knowledge exists as such only in the moment of being validated by scientific means and absorbed into the purportedly universal corpus of scientific knowledge (1995, 430; 2002, 290).[5] The validation of indigenous knowledge, Agrawal further suggests, is a process fraught with power—one in which the bearers of indigenous knowledge are perpetually subordinated to the stewards of science, made to act as eyes and ears to a scientific brain (Howes and Chambers 1980, 327).[6] Despite attempts to shift the boundary of science to encompass traditional medicine within its domain, then, this maneuver entails the construction and maintenance of other boundaries between scientific knowledge and its dubious others—boundaries that traditional healers, by definition, fail to recognize but must nonetheless be made to respect. Because scientific knowledge and its categorical others must be held separate even while the borders that define science allow the passage of indigenous knowledge from one side to the other, the exterior space of tradition must be constantly "sanitized" (Stirrat 1998, 242) as a site of "purified" production. Bearers of indigenous knowledge in its raw form must be quarantined in this space—kept well away from the border where they and their knowledge might be "polluted" and/or where they might act as gatekeepers, usurping the borderland brokerage of indigenous knowledge over which stewards of science claim exclusive dominion.

Hence, while policymakers and health officials in postwar Mozambique have been prepared to celebrate the indigenous knowledge of traditional healers and to draw upon it as a resource in the neoliberal climate of state decentralization and economic austerity, they have not been prepared to conceive of traditional healers fully as colleagues, whether in the realm of medical research or health care. To do so would be to undermine their status as the authoritative guardians of vital therapeutic knowledge and resources. Indeed, to do so would be to jeopardize their very claim to modernity—a claim that even after the demise of FRELIMO's project to bring about socialist modernization in Mozambique necessitates a traditional other and a boundary with which to sustain the divide.

Notwithstanding the indigenous knowledge paradigm animating health policy reform in post-socialist Mozambique, however, my findings suggest that the knowledge, and the power, of so-called traditional healers is inextricably bound up with *their transgressions of* boundaries between categories such as "indigenous" and "scientific," "traditional" and "modern." The healers with whom I worked in Mueda situated themselves at borders between the traditional and the modern, between the indigenous and the scientific, between the familiar and the foreign, between the local and the global, between this world and a dimly perceived other world, and even between good and evil, (re)drawing these borders in the act of managing flows across them. Like their "colleagues" of official standing in the national health service, these healers acted as brokers of the therapeutic resources within their grasp. Indeed, even as traditional healers' advocates sought to vouchsafe the value and integrity of their indigenous knowledge, these so-called traditional healers worked assiduously to transcend the bounds of locality, of indigeneity, and of tradition with which these sympathetic reformers circumscribed them. Their legitimacy *as traditional healers*, in fact, generally depended upon such border work.

Terezinha "Mbegweka" António

My research collaborators[7] and I spent considerable time in 1999 with the healer Mbegweka, who also served as assistant president of AMETRAMO for Mueda District. On the night of August 1, our work with Mbegweka culminated in our passing the night in her compound in Mueda town as she presided over a healing ceremony for a woman having difficulties nursing her newborn child. The woman's breasts were greatly engorged—each one was nearly as large as her head. When her child suckled, she had reported to Mbegweka, her breasts did not let down milk. She had lost her previous child because she was unable to nurse it; she feared that she would lose this one as well.

On the preceding day, Mbegweka had asked Marcos Mandumbwe and I to take her nephew with us as we traveled outside of Mueda town to conduct interviews in a nearby village. According to her instructions, we had dropped the youngster along the way in the village of Mpeme and fetched him on the return trip. By that time, he had organized a small troupe. They carried several drums, which they would play for Mbegweka's healing rite. When we arrived in her compound late the following afternoon, we found the place transformed. From a pole driven into the ground in the center of the yard flew a flag adorned with a red crescent and star above Arabic script. Two fires burned at the edge of the yard around which the young men we had brought the day before heated drum skins.

Once darkness settled, the drumming began. The ritual more closely resembled the healing practices of *ngoma* (Janzen 1992; van Dijk, Reis, and Spierenburg 2000a) or *zār* (Boddy 1989, 125–165) healers than the methods of other Makonde healers we had witnessed—healers who generally worked with *mitela* (medicinal substances) and the occasional incantation but not with drumming and dancing. Mbegweka led the patient out of the small closed pavilion in which she kept her *mitela* and seated her at the base of the flagpole. She then came to greet us, explaining that they would dance tonight to help the woman receive the spirit that afflicted her. Once the woman learned how to host her *jini*, Mbegweka told us, she would be able to nurse her child.

When Mbegweka stepped away, Marcos leaned close to me and said, simply, "*majini*" (pl.). Like me, he was struck by Mbegweka's use of the term—prevalent among Swahili populations on the Tanzanian coast, but foreign, and unfamiliar, to most Mozambican Makonde.[8] Mbegweka, we knew from previous conversations, had never been to Tanzania. Born in Palma (Cabo Delgado, Mozambique) in 1949, her parents had baptized her Terezinha António when she was born. "I was never given a Makonde name," she told us, "but the name I use in my healing practice is Mbegweka"—a name we later learned meant "I am alone." Mbegweka's parents both died while she was young—of what, she did not tell us. She passed the years of the Mozambican war for independence (1964–1974) in a zone controlled by FRELIMO in the Imbuho lowlands east of the Mueda plateau. Rather than returning after the war to the Palma region, where she "had

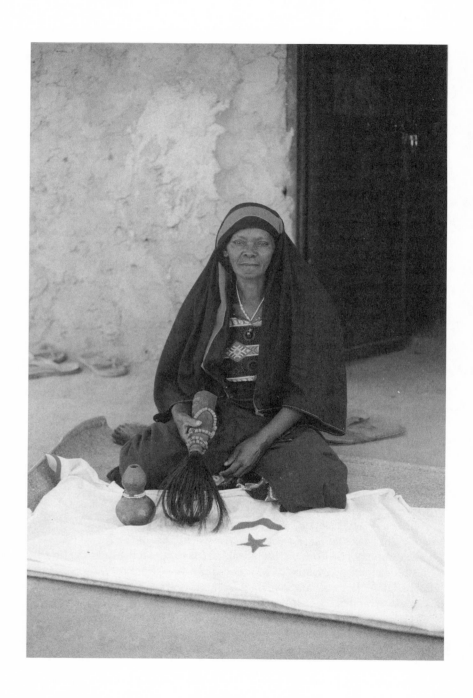

no one," she moved to Mueda town. Around this time, she told us, she fell ill. She was taken to an *nkulaula* (healer) who attempted to cure her, but her illness persisted. Eventually she was told that she was possessed by a spirit. She explained to us:

> In the past, this kind of affliction—being possessed by spirits—was called *mangonde*. But in my case it was something special. I went to see my father's elder brother [a man named Libata], who was also an *nkulaula*. He told me that the spirit possessing me was my mother's father, Ndonagwamba Shing'oma, who had been a powerful diviner. These kinds of spirits—the spirits of ancestors—are called *vanungu*. In the past, when a person was possessed by this kind of spirit, she would get fevers and begin to tremble. Then the ancestor would ask her to perform a ceremony. Once she did this, it was finished. Nowadays, it's different. These spirits stay with you. They return again and again. Ndonagwamba left no successor when he died, so he was calling me to follow him. I started treating patients around 1978 or 1979. I learned my *mitela* from my uncle.

From that time onward, Mbegweka was guided in how to use her *mitela* by the spirits that possessed her, including Ndonagwamba. She was possessed by other ancestors on her mother's side, and then on her father's—all of whom helped her to decipher the afflictions of patients who came to see her. Eventually, she came to be possessed by spirits that her patients—and even she—considered exotic.[9]

"Recently, I have been possessed by spirits that come to me from Tanzania," Mbegweka had told us. "They live in caves there, in a region filled with wild animals. It is a very dangerous place.[10] Lots of Tanzanian healers go there to consult these spirits, but I have been fortunate; they come to me, here." She had punctuated her previous accounts by telling us: "I am waiting to be authorized to go there myself some day soon. I am waiting for the healers there to tell me that the spirits have authorized my visit."

In any case, soon after Mbegweka began to treat her own patients, she embraced Islam—a religion strange to most Muedans, who know of it only from their travels to the Cabo Delgado coast (whose Mwani and Makua populations are predominantly Muslim) or to Tanzania (whose Makonde people are mostly Muslim). The Christian-born Terezinha, who had attended school for only one year (in a FRELIMO bush school during the independence war) took the Muslim name Atija and began study in an Islamic school in order to learn to read.

It was the subject of this complex biography who now orchestrated "traditional healing" rites in her compound before us. As we looked on, Mbegweka led a dozen women out of her house. As they seated themselves in a circle around the pole, she stepped close to us once more to continue her quiet narration of the proceedings over which she officiated. These women, she explained, were also patients under her care, each one learning to work with the *jini* spirit that possessed her.

Mbegweka took her place in the circle as the women began to sway with the rhythm of the drums. The tempo steadily increased until the women's upper bodies thrashed forcefully to and fro. In time, the women rose and began circling the pole. The drums beat out a frantic tempo as the women raced around the flag. When they slowed—as they did from time to time—two or three of the women would begin grunting and snorting, eventually falling on the ground in a state of hysteria somewhere between laughter and sobbing. They were summoning their "Arab spirits," Mbegweka reported to us, asking if we did not recognize this by the cutlasses the women brandished.[11] Indeed, the women menaced one another—as well as onlookers—with *catanas* (the Mozambican term for machetes).

Deeper into the night, the rhythm of the drums changed noticeably. Mbegweka passed by to tell us that the women were now summoning their "Makonde spirits." As she spoke with us, one of the women lunged from the circle toward a fire burning at the side of the yard, scattering bright orange coals and sending the drummers who huddled around the fire reeling. She was pulled away but left lying prostrate on the cold ground, weeping, for more than a quarter of an hour, after which she arose and slowly approached the fire once more. The assembly—with onlookers now numbering more than fifty people—closed around her as she stepped on the hot coals, extinguishing them one by one with her bare feet.

As I observed the scene before me, I worried that my amazement might somehow disrupt an enactment of "tradition" which those around me considered ordinary, even routine. I consciously averted my gaze from fellow onlookers for as long as I was able before quickly peeking out of the corners of my eyes at those around me. To my surprise, they appeared more astonished than I. Conversing with them later, I discovered that many were most taken by the "Arab spirits" that possessed Mbegweka's troupe.

As I watched the women in Mbegweka's troupe hosting their Arab *majini* spirits—and most of the women had never traveled farther than the lowland water sources at the plateau's edge from which they fetched water—my mind's eye wandered over the plateau landscape, across the Rovuma River border, settling somewhere in an ill-defined, dangerous, cave-filled region of Tanzania to which I had never been but from which Mbegweka had told us her *majini* came. In the midst of Mbegweka's compound, Muedans too—participants and observers—experienced a foreign land, at once enchanted and frightening, filled with powerful spirits from places most had never seen and of which many had never heard.[12] Mbegweka drew her force from other entities in distant temporal, geographical, and/or cosmological domains. Her power as a "traditional healer" lay not in rote learning and mastery of Makonde "tradition" but in her novel capacity to broker and apply powers derived from other times and places. Her knowledge as a healer lay not only in locally harvested *mitela*, but also in her ability to mediate between the here and now of her compound—a world familiar and accessible to her clients—and an exotic world instantiated within the space of the familiar in the moment of her healing rites.

Asala Kipande and Luis Avalimuka

Asala Kipande was another ranking AMETRAMO healer who resided in the town of Mueda. Kipande did not work with healing spirits, as did Mbegweka. Like her, however, he had converted to Islam. "Most *vakulaula* are not Muslim," he told us, "but there is a growing tendency these days for *vakulaula* to become Muslim." He had learned to read and write, he told us, so that he might be able to "interpret" the Koran to his patients—most all of whom professed to be Christian.[13]

Kipande *had* traveled to Tanzania. His travels, in fact, permitted him to boast an "international practice."[14] He proudly told us when we met with him that he had been to Tanzania the previous year and had joined a Tanzanian association of healers while there. As evidence of his claim, he produced for our inspection a receipt in the amount of 500 shillings for payment of dues to an organization called TAMOFA (The Tanzania Mozambique Friendship Association).[15]

Kipande fashioned himself a "traditional healer" who practiced "modern medicine."[16] He specialized in treating illnesses related to sexuality. He told us that many of his patients were men suffering from impotence. The most common problem he saw, he told us, was that of men who had had sex with prostitutes.

He explained:

> When menstrual blood gets inside a man's penis, it causes impotence. Normally, this doesn't happen. Most women have shame; they do not have sexual relations with their husbands when they are menstruating. The trouble is that prostitutes have no shame. They are concerned only with money, so they will have relations with a man while they are menstruating. And that can make the man impotent.

Kipande also treated female patients who suffered from what he called "blockage of the vaginal canal." He was proudest, however, of his ability to treat the diseases that he had heard his "colleagues at the hospital" refer to as "sexually transmitted diseases"—syphilis, gonorrhea, and AIDS.

When the topic of STDs arose in a conversation we had with him one day in his compound, Kipande stepped inside the small pavilion that he used for healing and reemerged with a shoebox. He opened it and pulled out a strand of JeitO condoms, the brand then being distributed throughout rural Mozambique by an NGO concerned with HIV education and prevention (Agha, Karlyn, and Meekers 2001; Karlyn 2001). He told us, matter-of-factly: "I give my patients one of these to use"—leaving us to wonder if a single condom might, according to Kipande's instructions, be used multiple times or instead if its one-time use might somehow be thought subsequently to "protect" its user against future perils.[17]

More important—as if in fulfillment of the prophecies of some celebrants of indigenous knowledge—Kipande told us that he knew how to cure AIDS. He

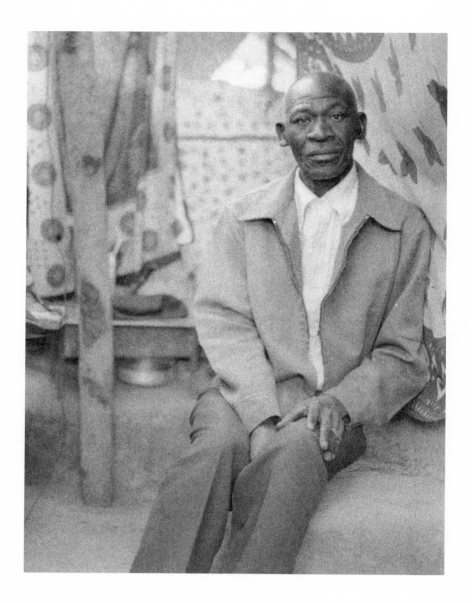

explained that he knew of a small tuber essential to the cure. He squeezed the pinky finger of his right hand at its first joint between the thumb and first finger of his left hand to show us the size of the tuber. "When you boil it, a red juice comes out," he told us. "You put that juice in a bottle and shake it well every day. People with AIDS should drink some of that juice each day. They will begin to urinate a lot—red foamy urine. AIDS passes out of them with that urine."[18]

I asked Kipande if he could supply me with a specimen of the root. He told us that he could not reveal his secret, but he assured us that his cure was effective.[19] He had already healed three people afflicted with AIDS, he declared. "One woman from Ndonde had tested positive for AIDS before coming to see me," he said. "After my treatment, she was tested again, and this time the test was negative."[20]

Among the other procedures Kipande performed were "vaccinations." While sitting in the compounds of other Muedan healers—who "vaccinated" clients for everything from bodily aches to persistent or recurrent illness to protection against sorcery attacks—I had witnessed treatments similar to the one Kipande told us he regularly performed. The procedure entailed making a series of cuts in the skin around the vulnerable or afflicted area of the body. The instrument used was a common razor blade. In the incisions, healers smeared *mitela*—generally made of burned and pulverized leaves, bark, and/or roots but often also containing acid extracted from a disposable battery.[21] "Vaccination"—to the frustration and horror of Kipande's "colleagues" at the hospital in Mueda—constituted one of the most common practices undertaken by Muedan *vakulaula*. As blades were used on dozens of patients without any attempt to sterilize them, hospital personnel feared that "vaccination" served as a vector for the transmission of hepatitis, if not the HIV virus.

Just before I left Mueda at the end of my research stint in 1999, Kipande requested that I bring him two items when I next returned to the plateau. The first was razor blades, the second was latex gloves. When I asked him why he needed these things, he told me that he feared contaminating his patients by using the same blades again and again and that he feared contracting diseases in the course of his work by getting his patients' blood on his hands. Clearly Kipande had been "reached" by public health educators.[22] I knew that inexpensive razor blades were readily available in the Mueda market; if he could not afford to buy enough of them to use a new one on each patient, he might have easily required each patient who came to him for "vaccination" to bring his or her own blade.[23] In time, however, it became apparent to me that Kipande wanted better-quality razor blades than could be found in the local market. Such quality "instruments" would set him apart from his *vakulaula* competitors. Similarly, latex gloves constituted a component of a more official "uniform" that would enhance Kipande's credibility with potential clients.[24] Already one of the most respected and visited *vakulaula* in Mueda, Kipande wished to consolidate his practice by upgrading his professional identity to "traditional doctor." Doctors—both he and his patients knew—wore gloves.[25]

Luis Avalimuka—another AMETRAMO healer living in Mueda town—also studied and replicated practices he witnessed in an official health care setting.[26] Luis worked with the aid of ancestors who visited him in dreams and directed him to the medicinal substances appropriate to the needs of his clients. When I asked him to tell me about recent cases that he had successfully treated, he ducked inside his house and reemerged with a school student's notebook. He put it on the table in front of us, the back cover facing up with print upside

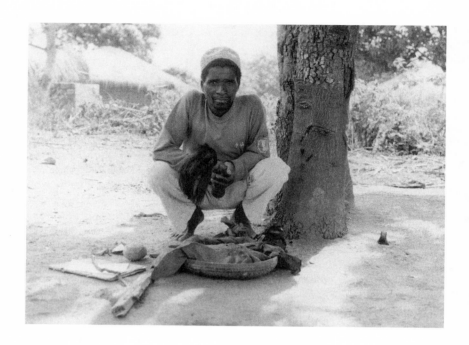

down. He opened the notebook, revealing a list of names. It was his "patients' register," he told us.[27] The first entry was dated August 18, 1991. He had begun keeping the register, he informed us, when he was instructed to do so in a dream. He turned the pages. The entries were numbered up to 230, and several dozen unnumbered entries appeared at the end. He pointed out columns that indicated follow-up treatments and reports from patients on the treatment's success. I counted fifty-four successful treatments among the first 230 entries—a decent rate of success, I thought, when adjusted for patient noncompliance with treatment and for survey nonresponse.

Like Mbegweka, Asala Kipande and Luis Avalimuka were among the plateau's most widely respected and commercially successful traditional healers. Their success was inseparable from the fact that they did not idly await researchers from the Ministry of Health, or elsewhere, to validate their knowledge and harvest their medicinal substances and techniques into the stores of medical science. They scoured their world at its margins in their attempts to expand their knowledge, demonstrating creative disregard for the boundaries that others drew between "traditional healing" and "modern medicine." Indeed, their power as healers depended upon their transgressions of these boundaries. Whereas Mbegweka drew power from the geographical and cosmological borderlands that separated her from, and connected her to, her clients, rendering specious the description of her practices as "indigenous" or "local," Asala Kipande and Luis Avalimuka aggressively stretched—and sometimes openly spurned—the category of "traditional healer." Their healing repertoires incorporated practices that certainly were *not* "handed down from generation to generation . . . from time immemorial," as the World Health Organization defines "traditional medicine" (1978, 8). Neither was their disposition "traditional" in the sense of antimodern. These *vakulaula* enthusiastically inhabited whatever margins of the "official" world of medical "science" they found accessible.

AMETRAMO healers such as Asala Kipande and Luis Avalimuka were quick to point out that their association's registry was housed in the offices of the District Directorate of Culture, in the same building as the FRELIMO Party district headquarters. Prior to AMETRAMO's formation, the Cultural Directorate had begun registering healers in Mueda to keep tabs on them, but as the neoliberal state displayed less and less interest in overseeing their activities, these healers clung to their tenuous ties with patron-officials from whose recognition they derived legitimacy. Many *vakulaula* with whom we worked displayed government-issued documents for clients to see, just as medical doctors hang framed diplomas on the walls of their treatment rooms. Muedans healers such as Asala Kipande and Luis Avalimuka encouraged people to associate them with the institutions and practices of modern health care in accordance with their convictions that such associations enhanced their credibility *as traditional healers* (Green 1996, 24) and augmented their healing power. Through their boundary transgressions, these *vakulaula* redrew the lines that divided local from global, traditional from modern, and *kulaula* (healing) from biomedicine, situating themselves as gatekeepers between worlds known and unknown, accessible and inaccessible, to their clients. Notwithstanding reformers who sought to circumscribe them within the domain of traditional healing, these healers drew force from mediating categorical interstices of their own invention—borders they embodied in their innovative healing practices.

Julia Nkataje

AMETRAMO's network had not yet reached as far as the village of Namande when we visited Julia Nkataje at her home there in 1999. Even so, Julia's healing practice was perhaps the most frequented on the Mueda plateau. Her compound was a far busier place than the market in the center of the village. Within the boundaries of the bamboo fence that delimited her property, more than a dozen people rested in scattered patches of shade, while almost twice as many attended to tasks around a large house under construction. All of these people, we were told, were patients—some in-patients who resided for days, weeks, or even months at a time in the eighteen-bed dormitory adjacent to Julia's house, others out-patients who came to see her by day and returned home at night. Those who were able labored for her in exchange for the care she provided. They would soon finish the second dormitory, she told us, pointing to the house under construction.[28] After surveying Julia's establishment, my research collaborator, Marcos Mandumbwe, pronounced it a "healing factory."

When Marcos and I first entered her compound, Julia invited us to share the shade with her beneath an open-air tin-roofed pavilion. As we spoke with her,

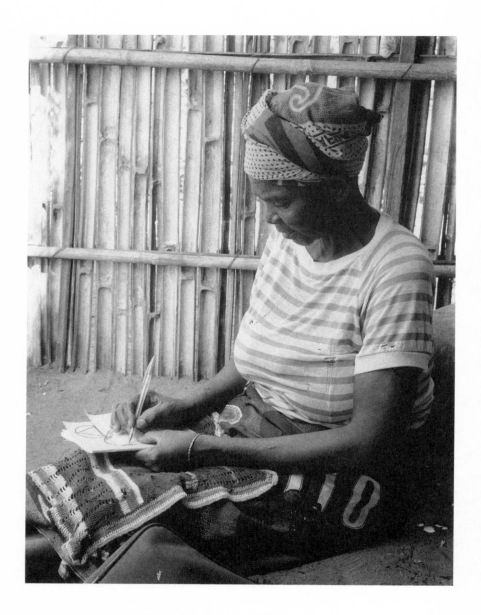

she sat with her back against one of the wooden poles holding up the roof. She rested a primary-school exercise notebook on her lap. With great deliberation, she used a blue ballpoint pen to draw what looked to me like curlicues on each line of a strip of paper torn from one of the notebook's pages. As we conversed, she focused her eyes on her drawing, never looking at us. I wondered at first if she doodled to alleviate anxiety produced by our visit, but I eventually learned otherwise.

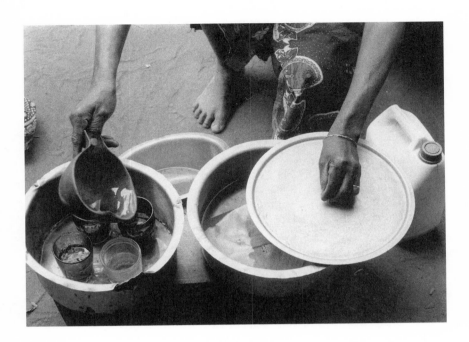

In response to our questions, Julia told us that her healing career began with her own illness soon after Mozambican independence. She suffered from headaches for more than three years. During that time, she told us, her body was always hot. Eventually, an *nkulaula* in the village of Miteda named Lapiki Madigida discerned that Julia's illness was due to sorcery. He did not reveal to her the identity of her attacker, but he cured her nonetheless. Once she was healed, she told us, she heard voices telling her to get a pen and paper. "The voices told me to draw these figures," she said, holding up a strip of paper. "They told me to put these writings in a pot of water and to boil them. Then, they told me to give the water to my mother to drink. She suffered from leg pains [a common symptom of sorcery attack] at the time, and the water cured her."

Thus began Julia's career as an *nkulaula*. As she later demonstrated for us, she regularly replicated the process she first used years ago to heal her mother. Patients came to her suffering from sore throats and headaches, from gonorrhea and HIV, from impotence and infertility. They sometimes suffered "God's illnesses" and they were sometimes the victims of sorcery. No matter, Julia told us, she healed them all the same. Whatever the affliction, she prescribed three glasses per day.[29]

From a recycled five-liter British Petroleum motor-oil jug, Julia poured water into cups. As she summoned her patients to approach, she told us that she was, in fact, a Christian. "The Virgin Mary has appeared to me four times," she said, in confirmation of this. The patients now lined up at the edge of the pavilion. As there were four cups, the patients were treated in groups of four. They kneeled

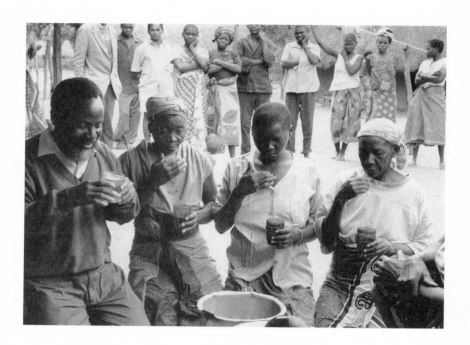

in front of the cups and picked them up. As they drank, together, they made the sign of the cross over their hearts.

I asked Julia what she wrote on the strips of paper. "*Sibila*," she told me.

I wondered if she took the term from the Portuguese "*sílaba*," meaning syllable. In any case, I associated her technique with accounts I had read of healers who used the pages of sacred texts like the Bible or the Koran in healing rites (Gray 1969, 175; Harries 2001, 420; Knipe 1989, 92; Obbo 1996, 190; Peletz 1993, 162; Rasmussen 2001b, 142; Shaw 2002, 253; Stoller 1989, 50; Whyte 1982, 2061; Whyte 1988, 225; Whyte 1997, 165). I later learned that Lapiki—the man who healed Julia—was Muslim and that he sometimes tore pages from the Koran, rolled them up, and placed them in a bottle that he gave to patients afflicted with mental illness. Lapiki, Julia told us, could not read the Koran. Julia was herself illiterate; what is more, she was not Muslim. Still, Julia's marks looked vaguely like Arabic script, even if she wrote from left to right.

I asked her about this. "It's not the Koran that I write," she told me.

"What is it, then?" I asked. "Does it have meaning?'

"Yes," she answered, confidently. Then she smiled softly, adding, "But *I* don't know what it means."

Whereas Julia's border work between the domains of Christianity, Islam, and Makonde "tradition" further challenges the notion that Muedan healers are the bearers of *indigenous* knowledge, Julia's response leads me to interrogate the other half of the phrase, indigenous *knowledge*, and the assumptions contained therein.

Medical anthropologist Byron Good (1994, 15–17) has argued—following Needham (1972) and Smith (1977)—that Western science displays unfounded arrogance in its assumption that *we* (scientific thinkers) *know,* while *they* (unscientific thinkers) only *believe.*[30] Muedans themselves would agree with the notion that *vakulaula* are the bearers of *knowledge* rather than mere *believers.* Indeed, when Muedans speak euphemistically of a healer, they describe him or her as one who "knows a little something" ("*kumanya shinu shoeshoe*"). The source of a healer's power lies precisely in what he/she *knows.*[31] In acknowledgment of the epistemological status of native thought, contemporary anthropologists generally use the term *knowledge* where once they spoke of their subjects' *beliefs* (Humphrey and Onon 1996; Kapferer 1997; Lambek 1993; Stephen 1996). It is a rhetorical move that advocates of indigenous knowledge enthusiastically affirm.

Paul Sillitoe has cautioned us, however, against plucking indigenous knowledge from its context and against assuming that we understand fully what others' knowledge is about (1998, 227–228).[32] Although the M.D.'s prescription is often every bit as "illegible" to his patients as Julia's script, Julia and the M.D. probably hold vastly different conceptions of writing as a form of knowledge. Roy Ellen has suggested that the assumption embedded within the indigenous knowledge paradigm that knowledge is empirical may occlude from view moments when knowledge is more a way of discovering and/or experiencing the world than it is data about the world (1998, 239). Such is often the case, I would argue, with Julia Nkataje's knowledge and that of her fellow Muedan *vakulaula.*

Indeed, what Muedan *vakulaula* "know," as Ellen predicts, is bound up with a distinctive way of seeing the world—a mode of envisioning the world that is inescapably associated with sorcery.[33] Muedan sorcerers, it is said, are able to see the world differently than ordinary Muedans. Theirs is a vision that allows them to gain decisive leverage on the world and thus to (re)make it in astonishing and often horrifying ways, producing illness and misfortune in those upon whose well-being they feed. Muedan healers are said to undo the ill effects of sorcery in their patients by, in turn, gaining decisive perspectives on those whose destructive attacks are otherwise invisible. *Vakulaula* are in fact assumed by Muedans to *be* sorcerers, for how could they see the destructive acts of sorcerers unless they were able to see as sorcerers see, to know as sorcerers know? The euphemism through which healers are often described is the same one generally applied to sorcerers: *"Aju, andimanya shinu shoeshoe!"* ("That one, he/she knows a little something!")

While Muedans invest confidence in the idea that the healers whom they consult use their knowledge to treat the ill effects produced by others, they look upon *vakulaula* with deep ambivalence, for not only do they traffic in the same substances as common predatory sorcerers, they also possess the power to wound, devour, and destroy—a power that finds expression even in their healing practices, which turn the effects of sorcery back upon those who have attacked their patients. While Muedans hope that their healers do not—or, at least, "no longer"—use their knowledge to feed their own wanton appetites, most remain unsure of this. The power of the healer, as most Muedans understand it, derives from the position he/she stakes in a borderland somewhere between creation and destruction, somewhere between good and evil. As healers mediate between the domains of healing and harming, beneficence and malevolence converge within their bodies. They work the border to beneficial effect, but the question remains: to whose benefit—their patients' or their own?

It is revealing that healers are said to know *only* "a little something." While healers depend on the popular assumption that they *do* know *something* and foster such convictions in various ways, most would themselves claim to know no more than "a little," for to possess unbounded knowledge would not only confirm suspicions that one knew the other side of the border between the visible and the invisible realms *too* well but would also invite attack by sorcerers keen to test one's true abilities.

Knowledge of the invisible realm of sorcery—which, among Muedans, is determinative of one's health and well-being—is in any case broadly understood to be inherently partial and inevitably tenuous. To know sorcery is to know that decisive forces are invariably capricious and unwieldy. As the healer Sinema Kakoli once told us, "Most who do battle in the realm of sorcery wind up losing in the end." Thus, what a prudent healer *knows* is as much about the *limits* of knowledge as anything else: not only is there always someone else who knows a little more—someone who poses a lethal threat to one's well-being—but the decisive logics of the world are, ultimately, unknowable to all. Knowledge conceived in this way resists instrumentalization as envisioned by the would-be harvesters of indigenous knowledge.

Julia did not know the meaning of the healing figures that passed through her hands and onto the paper before her. Through her healing practices, however, she inhabited the borderland between the knowable and the unknowable—a locale of vital interest to her afflicted clients. Indeed, for her clients, Julia embodied the border she mediated between certainty and doubt about the world's mysterious workings. It is ironic that in so doing Julia acted much like her biomedical "colleagues" at the hospital in Mueda—whether Mozambican or foreign— who exercised knowledge the operative logics of which often lay beyond their full comprehension. Where Julia admitted what she did not know, however, her biomedical counterparts were somewhat more reluctant to do. Such subtle differences lead many Muedans, who often refer to sorcery (and countersorcery healing) as "a science," to ask themselves just what kind of science sorcery is, meaning how it is in fact like and unlike—even how does it measure up to—the other "sciences" to which they have been exposed over the years (colonialism, socialism, development).

Perhaps the most important difference for Muedans lies in the fact that Julia and her fellow *vakulaula* worked the boundary not between the known and the unknown but between the knowable and the unknowable. By continuously (re)producing and calling attention to the domain of the unknowable, they not only differentiated themselves from biomedical practitioners but challenged the claims of science about its ability to unceasingly advance the frontier of knowledge. Some things, Muedans healers perpetually asserted through their various practices, were simply unknowable, no matter what kind of knowledge one possessed, no matter what kind of "science" one subscribed to. Those who claimed to know too much, *vakulaula* constantly reminded their clients, actually knew very little.

In any case, where the indigenous knowledge paradigm that has animated the Mozambican transition to a policy of liberal tolerance for traditional healers has conceived of healers' knowledge as bits of data for collection and insertion within a taken-for-granted epistemological framework, it has obscured a truth that holds in relation to all healers, whether they are categorized as "traditional," "modern," or somewhere in between, namely, that the power of healing lies in no small measure in an entrepreneurial maneuver (a "gnostic approach," as Bates [1995, 3] might call it), that emphasizes the knower over the known. Successful healers—and Mbegweka, Asala Kipande, Luis Avalimuka, and Julia Nkataje were among the most respected, most sought-after healers we encountered on the Mueda plateau—sometimes cross boundaries, sometimes ferry their clients back and forth between domains, and sometimes stand guard over impenetrable borders. Regardless, to their clients they embody the very boundaries they mediate between here and there, between then and now, between we and they, between good and evil, between knowable and unknowable, and, perhaps most important, between the possible and the impossible.

Notes

In addition to presentations made with and to the Healing Divides group at the November 2002 Meetings of the American Anthropological Association in New Orleans and at the African Studies Center at the University of Pennsylvania in January 2003, draft versions of this essay were also presented as papers at the University of Chicago African Studies Seminar, the Indiana University Anthropology Seminar, the School of Oriental and African Studies (University of London) Anthropology Seminar, the University College London (University of London) Anthropology Seminar, and the Sussex University Anthropology Seminar, where numerous people provided stimulating commentary. I wish to thank especially Andrew Apter, John Campbell, Gracia Clark, Jennifer Cole, Jean Comaroff, John Comaroff, Kit Davis, Matthew Engelke, Steve Feierman, Ellen Foley, Stacey Langwick, Charles Leslie, Tracy Luedke, Trevor Marchand, David Pratten, Lee Schoen, Tonya Taylor, Rijk van Dijk, Megan Vaughan, and Richard Werbner. With permission from The University of Chicago Press, passages have been drawn from a previous publication: *Kupilikula: Governance and the Invisible Realm in Mozambique* (© 2005 by The University of Chicago Press. All Rights Reserved.).

1. Semali (1986, 88) and Feierman (1986, 214) describe similar initiatives being undertaken in socialist Tanzania in the mid-1970s by the Traditional Medicine Research Unit at the University of Dar es Salaam.
2. Green (1994, 44–45) further argued that only minimal benefits could be de-

rived from bioprospecting of medicinal substances owing to the high cost of laboratory analysis and pharmaceuticals testing. See also Pearce (1986, 255) and Chavunduka and Last (1986). Cf. Posey (1990).

3. See also Stoller (1989, 171) for description of a similar phenomenon among Songhay in Niger.

4. Green's approach was by no means unique among medical anthropologists and ethnobotanists. Consider, for example, the work of Wade Davis, the famed Harvard ethnobotanist who in the early 1980s investigated reports of the existence of zombies in Haiti (1988). Davis took seriously Haitian legends suggesting that powerful *bokor* (Voudon priests) could raise the dead from their graves and keep them as zombie slaves. In the course of his research, Davis isolated pharmacological substances that he concluded were capable of producing the zombie effect as described in Haitian folk narratives. In doing so, he suggested not only that Haitian zombie beliefs were grounded in truth but also that the truth of this "indigenous knowledge" could—indeed, had to—be validated by Western science. See also World Health Organization (1978, 29). Cf. Plotkin (1993, 237), who expresses greater ambivalence regarding the scientific paradigm as a standard of verification, although he uses it as such in any case.

5. See also Ulluwishewa (1993).

6. See also Brouwer (1998).

7. Since initiating field research in Mueda in 1993, I have benefited greatly from the collaboration of Marcos Agostinho Mandumbwe. Eusébio Tissa Kairo also assisted in the research upon which this chapter draws.

8. Janzen (1992) gives detail about the role of *majini* spirits in healing practices on the East African coast. See also Boddy (1989, 143), who tells us that the *zayran* spirits that possess Hofriyati women are a class of *majini*. Cf. Willis and Chisanga (1999, 147n4), who provide account of the appropriation of the Kiswahili term *majini* by Lungu people in Zambia to refer only to "evil spirits."

9. When she spoke of the spirits of her own ancestors, Mbegweka used the Shimakonde term *mangonde*; when she spoke of the other spirits that eventually possessed her, she used the term *majini*.

10. M. Green (1994, 37) tells us that Pogoro healers in Tanzania often work with the aid of spirits who inhabit "pools of still deep water in a section of unviolated forest."

11. Boddy (1989, 284–288) reports that Hofriyati also classify some of the *zayran* who possess them as "Arab spirits."

12. Boddy (1989, 165) reports that Hofriyati *zayran* spirits also generally "originate in locales exotic to that of the village." Janzen (1989, 239–240) suggests that spirits of distant provenance have come to be regarded as increasingly more powerful in central and southern Africa.

13. See also Whyte (1982, 2057).

14. Azande witch doctors did this even in Evans-Pritchard's time (1929/1967, 18). Last (1992, 398) reports that among Nigerian Hausa, the value of "foreign" remedies is greater owing to their "strangeness." See also Whyte (1982, 2061).

15. To my knowledge, TAMOFA has no formal function in relation to traditional healing.

16. Or, Kipande considered himself more an "indigenous practitioner of modern medicine" than a "practitioner of indigenous medicine," as Taylor has put it (quoted in Whyte 1982, 2060).

17. Tracy Luedke (personal communication, January 5, 2004) provided stimulating commentary on the uses of condoms as "magic bullets" not only by rural Mozambicans but also by public health workers who fetishized condom distribution statistics in a manner ironically reminiscent of socialist-era central planners despite the fact that by many accounts a high percentage of condoms distributed were used as balloon toys by children.

18. African healers who claim to be able to cure AIDS are legion. See, for example, Probst (1999).

19. See also Forster (1998, 538).

20. At the time of our conversation, Mozambique did not yet have facilities for HIV testing even in Maputo. The few Mozambicans who wished to be tested and who could afford it generally traveled to South Africa to be tested.

21. White (1994, 363; 2000, 99) suggests that injections have long been the object of fear and fascination in Africa. Vaughan (1991, 59) suggests that this fascination gave rise to Africans assimilating the medical practices of Western missionaries into their healing repertoires. In any case, "vaccination" has become a common component of the repertoire of many African healers. (See, e.g., Ashforth 2000, 48, 116; Ashforth 2001, 213; Beattie 1963, 42; Davis 2000, 237; M. Green 1994, 37; Janzen 1989, 241; LeVine 1963, 235; Marwick 1950, 104; Redmayne 1970, 113; Whyte, van der Geest, and Hardon 2002, 112; Willis and Chisanga 1999, 138; Yamba 1997, 214–215.) Whyte (1982, 2060) makes specific mention of the use of battery acid in such healing practices in Uganda. See also Wafer (1991, 91) regarding similar practices in Brazilian *candomblé*.

22. According to Tracy Luedke (personal communication, April 17, 2002), AMETRAMO members in Tete Province participated in NGO-sponsored HIV awareness workshops that alerted them to the potential dangers of razor blade "vaccination."

23. I had witnessed "vaccination" clients take such precautions of their own accord. One of my research collaborators, who sometimes sought relief through "vaccination" for a recurrent backache, began taking this precaution after working for a stint as a public educator in an NGO-sponsored HIV awareness campaign in Pemba.

24. Langford (2002, 188–230) provides an interesting discussion of how an Ayurvedic healer with whom she worked enhanced his credibility among his clients through what she describes as the fetishistic deployment of objects and procedures associated with medical science. Luedke (personal communication, January 5, 2004) reports that the midwives with whom she worked generally insisted upon being photographed while displaying the shiny medical kits given them upon completion of their training course. Langford is quick to point out that biomedical practitioners often deploy objects in ways that might be similarly described as fetishistic. See also Chalmers (1996, 9) and Rekdal (1999, 471).

25. I prepared for field research by training as an emergency medical technician. In the emergency medical kit that I carried with me in the field were several pairs of gloves. When Kipande made his request, I promised myself that I would give him a pair before leaving. Over the next few days, I imagined

Kipande using and reusing the gloves—as I had sometimes seen health workers do in Mueda's hospital—turning them inside out once they had become "too soiled." I also imagined how these gloves might assist Kipande in assuring his patients that his "vaccinations" were sterile and safe, and I questioned whether I wanted to contribute to this impression. When I next saw him, Kipande had forgotten the requests that he had made of me, and I decided not to remind him.

26. Bongmba (1998, 176) tells of how Wimbum healers in Cameroon bottle and label their medicinal substances so as to make them attractive to a "modern" clientele. See also Simmons (this volume).

27. See also Dillon-Malone (1988, 1160), who describes the use of patient record books among healers in Zambia, and M. Green (1997, 320–321), who describes written records kept by witch-cleansers in southern Tanzania.

28. Redmayne (1970, 108) encountered similar healing compounds, replete with dormitories, in colonial Nyassaland.

29. Danfulani (1999, 190) reports that among Eggon healers in Nigeria, "holy water" is similarly administered for "all diseases." See also Ashforth (2000, 46), who tells of a South African healer who prescribed the same herbal concoction for all ills.

30. Good warns that the concept of belief, so easily attributed to others, is a distinctively Western one that has come to connote conviction to a given idea or principle within the modern context of (and despite) uncertainty. From the scientific perspective, Good tells us, "[k]nowledge requires both certitude and correctness; belief implies uncertainty, error or both" (Good 1994, 17).

31. Willis and Chisanga (1999, 117) tell us that the term commonly used in southern Africa for healer—*ng'anga*—literally means "knower." David Pratten (personal communication, October 19, 2004) reports that the term for diviner/healer in Ibibio, *abia idiong*, literally means "specialist of knowledge."

32. See also Nuttall (1998, 22).

33. I address this issue in greater detail elsewhere (West 2005).

2 Presidents, Bishops, and Mothers: The Construction of Authority in Mozambican Healing

Tracy J. Luedke

Healing, in whatever form, involves power: the power of possessing and deploying specialized knowledge, the power to vanquish the debilitating forces of illness and misfortune, the power to transform the body. In Tete Province, Mozambique, the power to transform individual bodies through healing is intimately linked to healers' abilities to (trans)form social bodies in their roles as the leaders of associations, churches, and social networks. Healers in Tete claim and enact leadership roles by both drawing on a broad range of culturally and historically modeled constructions of power and authority and erecting boundaries of acceptability and legitimacy around the collage of practices and procedures they have assembled. This chapter addresses the ways healers in Tete, Mozambique construct authority for themselves as leaders and for the groups they lead.

The particular cultural field on which the chapter focuses is a community of healers and healed in northern Tete Province who call themselves "prophets," or *aneneri* (*neneri* sing., *aneneri* pl., literally "one who speaks for another") in the local language Chinyanja. Practicing at the interface of religion and medicine, members of this community cure illness by means of their possession by Christianized spirits, which are understood to have been sent by God. The cross and the Bible are potent symbols and tools for prophets, as are the medicinal roots they use to treat illnesses. The healing practices of this community reflect the individual and collective historical experiences of residents of this region. *Aneneri* first appeared in Tete around 1993, just after the end of the war that raged in Mozambique between the government (FRELIMO) and rebel forces (RENAMO) from shortly after independence from the Portuguese in 1975 until a peace accord in 1992. During the war, approximately 70 percent of Tete's residents fled the violence and terror of the war for neighboring Malawi, Zambia, and Zimbabwe, many staying for as long as ten years (Azevedo 2002, 141). Residents who fled northern Tete for Malawi found that the language and many cultural practices were familiar, but Malawian culture also reflected its history as a British colony and site of Protestant Christian missionizing, which had engendered religious and healing practices which differed from those of Mozambique, with its history of Portuguese colonialism and the dominance of the Catholic Church. It was during their time as refugees that Mozambicans encountered the *aneneri*. When the war ended, Mozambican refugees flooded back into Mozambique, and many residents returned to Tete bearing what they had experienced. For those individuals in whom Malawian prophets had discovered healing spirits, these spirits, their knowledge, and the rites and bodily practices they require accompanied the refugees in their return to Mozambique at the end of the war. Since then, the community of prophets has continued to reproduce and is now large and vibrant in Tete Province.

Therapeutic Entrepreneurialism

The substance and form of the healing practices described here reflect the flow of knowledge, practices, individuals, and objects across various political and social boundaries, including national borders, the contours of political and religious institutions, and bodies of "traditional" and "modern" medical knowledge. But this border-crossing by people, ideas, and things and the creative production of new cultural forms that has accompanied it have not gone undisputed. Self-made leaders within this context expend considerable energy to erect new boundaries that might contain the cultural forms associated with healing. Through this process of transgressing and constructing boundaries, both leaders and followers attempt to make sense of and put order to an often-times unruly set of experiences, including experiences of suffering and dislocation which threaten to "unmake the world."[1]

The process of "remaking" or "making anew" the world, which is inherent to both prophetic healing itself and attempts of local leaders to control and order it, is marked by contradictions and ellipses. The disordering of individual and social lives by various historical and political forces has, on the one hand, produced the creative assembly of new cultural forms that would make sense of this cacophony of experiences. On the other hand, the possibilities afforded by this disorder have allowed individual actors to claim and wield power of their own construction. The legacies of abuse of power, through policy as well as through violence, and the aftermath of this abuse—flight and social disintegration—bear heavily on the populace, even in their absence, in the form of individual and social memory. And this environment allows ambitious individuals to construct and legitimize their own authority.

Several scholars have recently noted the role and meaning of "disorder" in postcolonial settings such as Mozambique. Desjarlais and Kleinman suggest that the endemic political violence characteristic of the "new world disorder," particularly that perpetrated in situations of civil unrest, in which violence comes, as it were, from every which way, engenders a state of "demoralization" or "moral entropy" (1994, 10) in the populaces that experience it. The region on which this chapter focuses has long been a site of violence at the hands of an array of both local and foreign actors, whose connections to one another and/or to greater unseen political forces have often been unclear to those who witnessed brutality on the ground. The chaotic aggression of these forces and the demoralization it has provoked have been answered with the ordering and "re-moralizing" acts of prophet healers as they construct new moral communities.

The work of these prophet healer-leaders can also be seen as an example of the "political instrumentalization of disorder" (Chabal and Daloz 1999, 141–163). That is, the would-be leaders of prophet networks, associations, and churches whom I discuss here do not just attempt to "make sense" of disorder but to capitalize on it. "Disorder," as Chabal and Daloz use it, refers to the modus operandi of the "informal, uncodified, and unpoliced" African political sphere, an "ordered disorder" which only seems disorganized to Western analysts who perceive in it dereliction or lack of system. In fact, entrepreneurial political maneuvering is long-standing and effective, as witnessed by the fact that Africa "works" (in a systematic way) not despite these seemingly disorderly elements, but precisely through them. Leaders, in this setting, build themselves by building constituencies accumulated through particularistic patrimonial relationships, interpersonal claims and investments.

Thus two important varieties of "disorder" inform the work of authoritative healers in Tete. The first is that of a particular moment of crisis produced by the political, economic, social, and military battles of recent Mozambican history. The second is a long-standing political sensibility in which leadership rests in the creative exploitation of social relationships of indebtedness and client-ship, vertical relationships between senior (leader, patron, expert) and junior (follower, client, adept). This is a domain which resists codification, locating power instead in particular personae and their abilities to discern and exploit boundaries, whether in terms of exclusion or inclusion. In the setting of contemporary Mozambique, these two dynamics of "disorder" dovetail, operating in tandem and instrumentally for healer-leaders. They are the push and the pull that draw constituents under the sway of particular prophetic healers, consti-tuting their power. As will be shown below, healer-leaders make use of both the fear born of crisis and the courting techniques of mentorship to draw adepts and followers into their circles of influence. Drawing on the historical experi-ences and cultural resources of the region, these healers are able to utilize both the breaking and the making of boundaries (around roles, techniques, and so-cial groups associated with healing) toward the construction of empowered po-sitionalities for their selves/groups.

Accounts of African healing and politics reveal the degree to which African healers operate as political actors. Some scholars note the link, especially among southern African healing cults, between "healing power" and "political power" (van Dijk, Reis, and Spierenburg 2000b, 6). Others note more generally the degree to which politics suffuses all aspects of African social life: "[A]ll politi-cal actors, from the political elites to the ordinary man and woman, share a common notion of the undifferentiated nature of the political which they all seek to employ profitably. . . . [I]t is the very nature of the political instrumen-talization of seemingly non-political issues which marks out the political in Africa. . . . [T]he boundaries of the political are unclear or, more accurately, very porous" (Chabal and Daloz 1999, 149). Bayart (1993) notes the significant role of "political entrepreneurs" in contemporary African politics. Drawing on a common set of tactics, these entrepreneurs operate at all levels of the social scale: the "small men," Bayart suggests, "also work hard at political innovation" (249) and are "frequently up-to-date with the stratagems of the 'big men'" (219). Further, these strategies and struggles are "the very stuff of political life" (211). I would suggest that the healer-leaders whom I address are good examples of this broadly defined political actor, the entrepreneur, whose position rests in a blurring of the boundary between individual and institutional power and who draws productively from this confusion.

In emphasizing the entrepreneurial maneuvers of healer-leaders I do not assume the primacy of individual actors or universally understandable "strategies" (as in rational choice theory). I suggest instead that political entrepreneurialism is a cultural category; the entrepreneur is produced in fact in the relationship between him/herself and his/her constituents, who also recognize and participate in this exchange. On the other hand, I would also not want to imply that the entrepreneur follows a cultural script. Indeed, in this cultural context, there is precedence placed on innovation and creative boundary-crossing, which is one of the characteristics that draws a constituency in the first place. The "therapeutic entrepreneurs" who are the prophet healer-leaders engage in unprecedented innovations and the transcendence of categories and boundaries even as their innovations and transcendence are anticipated if not expected.

The *neneri* healers and leaders whom I discuss in this chapter are examples of this kind of "entrepreneur." I attend especially to the ways these healer-leaders conceptualize and claim their authority and legitimacy and that of the institutions they construct. These conceptualizations vary in some respects among the three kinds of entrepreneurial healer-leaders—mothers, bishops, and presidents —that I discuss. They also have much in common, as all assert their claims from the interstices between order and disorder, between individualized and institutionalized power, between the established and the improvised, between medicine, religion, and politics. They can be viewed as three lenses on the same phenomenon. Indeed, as will be addressed later in the chapter, these three institutional approaches and their authors often interlace and overlap with one another.

Mothers and "Cults of Affliction"

On Wednesdays and Saturdays, Magdalena[2] receives patients at her hospital in Domue, near the Malawi border in the district of Angónia in Tete Province. The patients come with various complaints of suffering born of ill health and misfortune. They come to mark consultations with Magdalena's biblical spirits, Petro (Peter), Yohane Batisi (John the Baptist), Lazaro (Lazarus), Yesu (Jesus), and Magdalena (Mary Magdalene). These spirits' powers include the ability to see into the human body; locate and analyze the illness, source of misfortune, or spirit presence therein; and prescribe the appropriate plant-based medicines in response. On consultation days, besides new patients, there are always present a number of Magdalena's former patients. These are individuals who came to Magdalena for treatment at some point in the past and in whom she discovered the presence of spirits. In bringing forth these spirits and mentoring their hosts, Magdalena became their spiritual "mother" (and they her spiritual "children") and their status as "prophets" (*aneneri*) was realized. Magdalena's large group of spiritual "children" is also present at her hospital on Sundays, when she holds sessions at which the spirits are called forth through singing, dancing, and prayer, and at larger ceremonies at which animals are sacrificed and new tools of the trade or work spaces are dedicated. Her "children" are Magdalena's followers, and their ample presence at consultations, meetings, and ceremonies attests to her power and prolificity as a healer.

As this profile of Magdalena shows, there are clear constituency-building strategies within the prophet community. The primary political tool of *aneneri,* which is also the general mechanism by which the community is created and grows, is the ability of healers to discover *neneri* spirits in others, a characteristic which the *aneneri* share with a multiplicity of other "cults of affliction" that exist throughout the southern African region (see Turner 1968; Janzen 1992; van Dijk, Reis, and Spierenburg 2000a). The more prolific a healer is in discovering new spirits, the more influence and authority are created. This requires both receiving a large volume of clients and discovering spirits in many of them (as opposed to diagnosing their illnesses as resulting from something else).

The relationship between the healer and the individual in whom she discovers a spirit is understood in terms of mother and child. Thus, *neneri* healers build constituencies in a way which mirrors a constituency and influence-building strategy typical of African societies—that of producing or cultivating dependents. In many African contexts, wealth, prosperity, and influence are sought through social reproduction, through "producing oneself by producing people, relations, and things" (Comaroff and Comaroff 1991, 143). As has been observed by a number of scholars of Africa, accumulating "wealth in people" is the key to commanding resources and status (See Guyer and Belinga 1995; Moore and Vaughan 1994; Bledsoe 1980).

The word for mother (*mayi*) is used to describe the healer's relationship to those he/she mentors spiritually, even when the healer is male. This reinforces the sense that the discovery of spirits acts as the birthing of a new social being, or the birthing of an individual into a new social status and new set of relationships and obligations. The newly discovered spiritual "child" (*mwana*), having been created by his/her "mother," will now serve in her ongoing creation as a sign of and active participant in her work.

Successfully building a constituency of spiritual children is a means of differentiation among healers. The number of children healers claim varies widely, from none or a few to hundreds or even thousands, depending on an individual

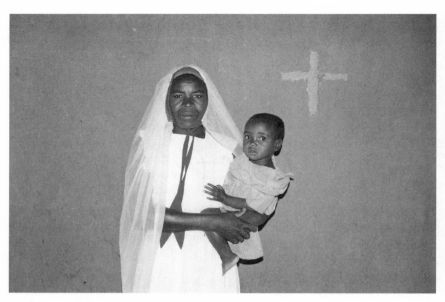

Estere, a prophet mother.

healer's longevity, popularity, and prolificity in discovering spirits. One index
(and a public display) of relative healer influence in this regard is the performance of spirit ceremonies.

The all-night ceremonies called by individual *aneneri* in the name of their
spirits are a site of enculturation into the *neneri* world, a place where key messages and bodily practices are publicly performed for a larger regional audience,
bringing diverse practices into at least relative synchrony. The ceremonies are
also an arena in which the politics of authority and leadership within the *neneri*
community are acted out and acted on. An individual healer's constituency (or
lack thereof) is physically manifested by means of the number of guests who
participate in his/her ceremonies, signaling how many children, patients, and
underlings owe allegiance to, or seek association with, that healer. For example,
I witnessed one spirit ceremony at the house of Magdalena at which at least 200
aneneri were present and another at the house of a relatively new and unknown
healer at which there were less than ten. At Magdalena's large ceremony, the
master of ceremonies was a prophet from Malawi who had traveled to Magdalena's home especially to fulfill this role. In fact, Magdalena had made a point
of inviting a number of *aneneri* from across the border. The long distances some
of these guests had traveled and the international nature (as well as the size) of
the crowd served as markers of Magdalena's status and influence, a display of
her symbolic capital.

The cultivation of a following, which acts as a symbolic resource in settings
such as the all-night ceremonies described here, also acts as a practical resource,
for example when the affairs of the *neneri* cult of affliction intersect with those

of the Association of Traditional Medicine of Mozambique (AMETRAMO). Besides her leadership role as a healer and mentor to other prophets within the social network of the "cult of affliction," Magdalena also leads other healers in the region in her role as the president of the traditional healers' association for the administrative post of Domue, a position which links her with the government (as will be further explained later in the chapter). Magdalena was elected to this position, many said, precisely because she has such a large following of "children" in the area, many of whom turned out for the elections and voted their "mother" into office. Magdalena capitalized on this position and sought to showcase it by using her position as a local leader of AMETRAMO to invite the government administrator for the locality (*chefe de posto*) to her ceremonies. On the second day of the two-day ceremony described above, several representatives of local government, including FRELIMO Party officials and schoolteachers, arrived in the stead of the *chefe de posto*. These guests, as representatives of the state, were offered to and received by participants as a sign of Magdalena's (officially recognized) status. The delegates reinforced this perception by making a formal statement to the crowd at the close of the ceremonies. Speaking for the *chefe de posto*, one of the schoolteachers stated that the *chefe de posto* knew the prophets were doing important work as healers, that they should continue with this work, and that the *chefe de posto* wanted to know about any difficulties they encountered. The crowd was then encouraged to present their problems or complaints as healers. Individuals stood and spoke of a variety of difficulties. Prominent among their complaints were references to the district-level president of AMETRAMO, a man named Gabrieli, including charges that he had harassed, extorted money from, and arrested and jailed *aneneri* and that he did not respect the leadership of their own local AMETRAMO president, Magdalena. Magdalena had in fact been troubled by ongoing conflict with Gabrieli. Their conflict came to a head when the president of Mozambique, Joaquim Chissano, made a rare visit to Angónia. The local administration called forth representatives of many community organizations and social groups to greet the president upon his arrival. Magdalena was invited by the FRELIMO Party to come as one of the leaders of the healers' association. But when Magdalena met up with Gabrieli in the district capital, he questioned her presence. She was only the president for Domue, whereas he was the president for the whole district, Gabrieli reminded her. What right did she have to greet President Chissano, especially without Gabrieli's permission? he demanded. He even grabbed Magdalena's clothes and shook her to make his point. The delegates promised to take these problems to the *chefe de posto* and have them resolved.

As the profile of Magdalena shows, spiritual mothering is a source of power that grows directly out of healing. It develops precisely through one's success as a healer, one's ability to attract patients, discover and draw out the spirits that trouble them, and mentor them in their roles as hosts to those spirits. Through this process healers accumulate constituencies of spiritual followers, a source of power that can be parlayed into other settings; for example, Magdalena's power as a "mother" afforded her influence with regard to AMETRAMO and the state. However, as Magdalena's experiences also attest, "mothering" is not the only means of power building available to prophet healers. Less transparent sources of power can be found in leadership positions linked to church and state which intersect with spiritual "mothering," at times buttressing and at times challenging its power.

Bishops and Churches

Yosefe is a *neneri* healer in Macanga District (Angónia's neighbor to the west) and the general bishop of Citizen Church, whose membership is composed of *aneneri*. He has recently completed construction of a large church building at his home near the district capital of Furancungo. As the bishop of Citizen, he is concerned to establish a link of support with white foreign missionaries who might legitimize Citizen and allow it to become an officially registered church, as he has seen happen with so many other local churches in Mozambique. The vice-bishop of Citizen is a woman named Mariya, a well-known healer who is much more active in this regard than Yosefe. She is also the founder of Citizen for the region of Macanga; as one of the earliest *aneneri* returnees to Macanga after the war, she was the first to establish a Citizen Church. Yet she enlisted Yosefe to act as the principle leader of the church because she felt it was necessary to have a man and a person who could read and write at the helm.

Mariya works as a healer by means of her *neneri* spirits, Mariya (Mary), Petro (Peter), and Yohane (John). Besides these spirits, she is troubled by another, a snake spirit who is the spirit of an ancestor on her father's side. The snake spirit causes problems for her, demanding, for example, that she smoke tobacco, which is prohibited by the *neneri* spirits, and disallowing her from having a husband or even sleeping with a man. As much as she has tried, however, she has not managed to expel the snake spirit, so she remains single and smokes at night, when her *neneri* spirits are distant.

The establishment of Citizen Church by Mariya and Yosefe, and indeed *neneri* activity throughout Angónia and Macanga, is but a recent chapter in the long history of Christianity in the region. From its very beginnings in the sixteenth century, Portuguese colonization of Mozambique included the presence of Catholic missionaries. The Jesuit Order of Catholic priests was particularly interested in the Zambezi Valley region, establishing residences there as early as 1610. In the late nineteenth and early twentieth centuries, formal missions were established at several sites within the province of Tete, including, in 1908, at Lifidzi in the district of Angónia. Jesuit historians wrote of Lifidzi: "We call Lifidzi a sign of hope. The climate is good, full of sun and plentiful rains which fertilize the land, abundant with corn, potatoes and every kind of vegetable and fruit. But the best thing of all is the people: kind, hospitable, and open to the word of God" (de Sousa 1991, 86). During the 1940s and 1950s, the Jesuits established at Lifidzi a large cathedral, residences for priests and nuns, dormitories for local boys and girls, schools, a maternity ward and dispensary of medicines, and workshops for the training of local men and women in carpentry, clothes making, and other trades. They also established further missions throughout northern Tete, including in Macanga in 1957. The Jesuit presence in northern Tete continued until the war forced the missionaries to flee in the late 1980s.

When the residents of Tete fled to Malawi, Zambia, and Zimbabwe during the war, they also came into contact with various Protestant and African Independent Churches that had established themselves in those countries and they encountered *aneneri* for the first time. In the period since the war ended and these refugees returned, Mozambique has seen a veritable explosion of missionary activity. As areas that had been dangerous became calm and with the increasing liberalization of government policy, a huge variety of both Western and African Christian denominations, arriving from North America, South America, and neighboring African countries, have spread throughout Tete. Thus, for much of the twentieth century, residents of northern Tete, even those who have not participated directly, have had ample contact with the symbols, objects, activities, and personae of Christian churches.

The *neneri* phenomenon generally reflects the process by which certain elements of Christianity have been taken up by local people, reinterpreted, and put to uses and ends that are often different from those they served in the context of the formal church. For example, the Bible is used as a tool in healing, crosses are sewn onto spirit uniforms, and the personalities of Bible stories appear as healing spirits. However, the degree to which *aneneri* have taken up the institutional form of the church has remained variable. In Angónia, the healing and religious activities of *aneneri* are organized around what are explicitly referred to as hospitals, whereas in Macanga, besides their healing activities, *aneneri* are also members of what are explicitly referred to as churches.

The lack of *neneri* churches in Angónia may reflect the greater and longer-standing Catholic presence in this area. The *aneneri* of Angónia all claimed to have been active Catholics in the past. They were forced to leave the Church, they said, with the arrival of their spirits, who prohibited them from attending. These *aneneri* explained that their spirits insisted on arriving during church services to reveal the illicit items, including amulets and witchcraft-related substances, that other members of the congregation or the clergy themselves possessed. The spirits' obsession with discovering and revealing these nefarious secrets in front of the congregation caused them so much trouble with the church fathers that they were forced to stop attending. The spirits also caused problems in church services because they cannot bear to be in close proximity to people who drink or smoke, as was the case with some members of the congregations. The spirits' obsessive moralizing against the most moralistic of communities— Catholic missionaries and their followers—seems like an ironic response to the rhetoric of the missionaries. It may be that the influence of the Catholic Church and people's identities as Catholics are strong enough, especially in the shadow of the large mission at Lifidzi, to stop them from forming or joining other kinds of churches. Even the *aneneri* who said they did not attend a formal church because of the above spiritual problems often still identified themselves as Catholics.

A more immediate reason that *aneneri* in Angónia have not organized explicit churches is the campaign waged in that district by Gabrieli, the president of AMETRAMO Angónia, against Citizen Church (described in greater detail in the next section). For Gabrieli, a key index of whether particular *aneneri* were law abiding or engaged in subversive activities was the architectural arrangement of a *neneri* healer's yard, specifically whether or not church and hospital were separated into two buildings. In fact, Gabrieli had several *neneri* healers arrested for convening their followers in a building that had been set aside as a church and was distinguished from the building where healing took place. Buildings, then, were understood to represent in material form conceptual distinctions or conflations between categories of social actors and activities.

In Angónia, *aneneri* operate out of one building, and this building is always explicitly referred to as a "hospital" (*chipatala*) or, more ambiguously, as a *kachisi*, a word meaning house of the spirits. This Chichewa word was originally used to refer to a house for sacrifices to or communications with ancestor spirits. The word was seized on by the translators of the Chewa Bible, who used it for the English word "temple." In a third incarnation, the word is now used by many *aneneri* to describe the house where both healing and praying takes place, the house in which the work of the spirits is performed. Even when what was happening inside the *chipatala* or *kachisi* was very much the same thing that happened inside a *tchalitchi* (church), *aneneri* in Angónia were loath to call it such.

In the neighboring district of Macanga, however, where Yosefe and Mariya reside, in addition to their healing activities, *aneneri* are members of churches. Healers in Macanga usually have two separate buildings in their yards, one a hospital for healing activities and the other a church for religious services and activities. There is little difference between what the *aneneri* of Angónia and the *aneneri* of Macanga do, but the symbolic significance of separation or unification of the various categories of activity in the same or different spaces signals a difference in the organizational models in place among the *aneneri* of the two zones.

One difference the institution of "church" precipitates in Macanga is that it allows for a different kind of leadership politics. In the context of spiritual "mothering," leadership emerges organically through the process of healing individuals and mentoring them as spirit hosts. Only successful healers are in a position to become leaders within this system. Many of these leaders are women, since the majority of the participants in the *neneri* community in general are women. In Macanga, however, where the institution of Citizen Church is bound up with *neneri* activity, leadership takes another form, based on that found within other kinds of churches. Thus, in Macanga one finds "bishops" and "reverends" arranged hierarchically over groups of *aneneri*. The bishops and reverends, although ostensibly healers, are often only nominally so and they are always men, despite the predominance of female healers and participants.

Women healers within Citizen still gain recognition, influence, and a certain amount of informal power, but they are not and cannot be bishops. This is the case for Mariya, who, although she founded Citizen Church in Macanga after the war and although she is a well-established and active healer, bears the title of vice-bishop, whereas the title of bishop rests with Yosefe.

The usurping of the organic leadership positions of accomplished women healers by men within Citizen is often effected by means of literacy.[3] The reading of Bible passages is a common demand of *neneri* spirits and requires that a somewhat literate person be on hand to read the chosen verses. Although the majority of the population, both men and women, is nonliterate, those who are literate are much more likely to be men. In Angónia, successful women healers will sometimes keep a literate male follower as an assistant in matters of reading. In Macanga, the role of the literate male assistant has been institutionalized in positions of power within the church structure. The gendered pattern of literacy and the model of male authority in other kinds of Christian churches have allowed men to claim positions of leadership within an otherwise female social phenomenon. Male *aneneri* in Macanga, as readers and leaders, have institutionalized a particular gendered model of authority.[4]

The power dynamics within Citizen Church are also not a closed system; they intersect with those of AMETRAMO and in turn the state. Yosefe, general bishop of Citizen Church, is also the president of AMETRAMO for the district of Macanga. While he feels that his role as bishop and the organization of Citizen Church are solid and growing, Yosefe is more concerned about his role as president of AMETRAMO. In 1995, Pedro Dos Santos, one of the provincial-level leaders of AMETRAMO, came from the city of Tete to Macanga to organize the local chapter of the association and appointed Yosefe as the district-level president. But since that time, there has been no further contact with or visits from the office in Tete, and Yosefe has had trouble maintaining the association. In particular, he has found it difficult to get healers to pay their membership dues, which he is supposed to send to the provincial-level fiscal officer in Tete, Manuel Olímpio. Yosefe finds that when he makes the rounds to collect dues, healers flee at his approach or deny that they are healers.

Thus, the *neneri* leadership positions associated with church and state bear varieties of power with their own complications. Whereas the power of the "mother" is born of and embedded in dense social networks, the authority of the bishop rests in assumptions about gender, literacy, and the practice of Christianity, assumptions that might be refigured or resisted.

Presidents and Associations

Gabrieli lives in Ulongue, the district capital of Angónia. Although he has a number of spirits and can cure many diseases, much of his time is taken up with organizational work and campaigns instead of with receiving patients. In addition to his role as district-level president of AMETRAMO, he is an active member of FRELIMO. He takes these two roles very seriously and perceives

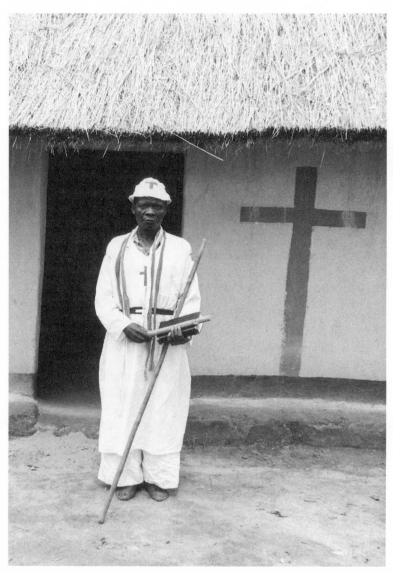

Yesu, a prophet healer and leader of Citizen Church.

them as linked. In recent years, two of his biggest preoccupations, against which he has waged fierce campaigns, have been witchcraft and renegade churches. In the late 1990s, he launched a major offensive against witchcraft during which he traveled throughout the district vaccinating members of rural communities. A second campaign which has occupied Gabrieli more recently is an offensive to eradicate from the district the prophetic healing church called Citizen, which

Gabrieli considers a front for the dissemination of propaganda by the opposition political party RENAMO. He has made several strikes against this church and its leaders and has had several people jailed for activities associated with Citizen. He considers all the work he does as a healer and as the president of AMETRAMO as "service to the government."

Gabrieli is but one local node in the hierarchy of AMETRAMO, the national professional organization of Mozambican traditional healers, which was officially recognized and registered by the government in 1992 (see West, Pfeiffer, this volume, on the history and operation of AMETRAMO). The advent of AMETRAMO reflected a change in the government's reactions to and dealings with traditional medicine. The ruling FRELIMO Party was born in the early 1960s as a radical response to the long and oppressive era of Portuguese colonialism. FRELIMO took power in 1975, armed with the ideologies and policies of Marxist-Leninist scientific socialism that had inspired and informed the independence struggle. Primary in this ideology was the need to banish all that was "backward" and "obscurantist" and thus contrary to the project of constructing the new society. In terms of traditional medicine, according to the main news magazine produced in Maputo in the early post-independence period, this meant that "we should effectively liquidate the superstition associated with traditional medicine, but take advantage scientifically of all that is positive within the popular Mozambican pharmacopeia" (da Silva 1975, 58). The official ideology of the times saw in traditional medicine both "good" and "bad" elements and strove to isolate and recuperate the "good."

This divide between the perceived positive and negative aspects of traditional medicine took several forms. One was the distinction between those traditional healers whose work focused solely on the application of medicinal plants and those whose work relied on spirits. The latter category was considered particularly insidious: "[T]his type of healer takes advantage of people influenced by obscurantist concepts, in order to deceive them with a series of mysteries. . . . The main question is how to educate the peasants scientifically in order to neutralize completely any possibilities for activity on the part of these exploiters" (Castanheira 1979, 12). The government's policies also reflected a desire to separate the medicinal plants themselves from the sociocultural context in which they were used. Toward this end, in 1977 the Cabinet for the Study of Traditional Medicine was formed as a subsection of the Ministry of Health. Its explicit goal was the study of the bioactivity of medicinal plants, removing to the laboratory what had until then had its place in the social life of the rural village.

FRELIMO's socialist ideology and policies shifted with time, as much in response to the pressures of poverty and the wielding of structural adjustment policies by political entities more powerful than itself as to any change of political heart. By the late 1980s, then, Dona Banú Idrisse Abdul, the founder of AMETRAMO and president until 2000, was in a position, if not to receive outright support from the government in her endeavors, at least to pursue openly her goal of creating an association of traditional healers. Dona Banú decided to organize the Association of Traditional Medicine of Mozambique in 1989 to provide a context for the exchange of knowledge and experiences among traditional healers. She traveled long distances from her home in Maputo at the southern tip of Mozambique to the provincial capitals to organize chapters of AMETRAMO and within a few years was able to establish a network. One of her first acts in establishing the association was to appoint a leadership hierarchy. In August 1992, AMETRAMO held its first "national conference" in Maputo, at which the directors of the National Executive Committee were elected, including Dona Banú as president, two vice-presidents, and a secretary-general. By the next month, each province had its own provincial president and vice-president and the bureaucracy grew from there. Soon there were also fiscal officers, treasurers, and various other bureaucrats in place to run the organization.

FRELIMO still has no explicit policy regarding traditional medicine, unlike neighboring countries which have active associations and have established hospitals of traditional medicine (for example, see Chavunduka 1986 on Zimbabwe). Despite FRELIMO's resistance to or indifference regarding traditional medicine, AMETRAMO is now closely associated with FRELIMO and the government, and the two entities share the same space in laypeople's understandings of the formal political structures that have jurisdiction over them. In Tete, and in other provinces as well, AMETRAMO has been given space for its office at FRELIMO's party headquarters. The AMETRAMO office in Tete is far from luxurious—it is located in the yard attached to the party offices, an area which also serves as a mechanics' garage for party vehicles—but it serves an important symbolic role. The office means that AMETRAMO is "recognized" by FRELIMO. And for many, including the officers who oversee the organization, it is a part of FRELIMO and is "doing the government's work." AMETRAMO also owes its political style to the culture of bureaucracy that has characterized the rule of FRELIMO (witnessed by AMETRAMO's hierarchical organization, which resembles those of other government entities), which was informed in turn by the model of the Portuguese colonial government. FRELIMO posters adorn the walls of the AMETRAMO office in Tete, and the policies and procedures that emanate from that office bear the mark of FRELIMO's bureaucratic style.

From the beginning AMETRAMO was rife with power struggles, fissions, and accusations of wrongdoing. The hierarchically organized financial system of the association, through which dues collected in the districts were to be sent to the provincial offices and then to the national office, never functioned as it was meant to. For the most part, dues never made it past the provincial level. There were cases of outright fraud in which local leaders reproduced membership cards and sold them off the record for their own profit. There were power struggles over who exactly was the designated president, vice-president, fiscal officer, and so forth. In 2000, there was a coup within AMETRAMO when a contingent of its leaders from southern Mozambique accused Dona Banú of diverting funds from the association and held their own "elections" in which they named a new national president. The supposed new leaders took out ads in the national newspaper claiming that Dona Banú had been ousted. Dona Banú fought back and filed a court case claiming defamation of character against those who accused her. In 2001, she and some of her supporters within AMETRAMO formed a new association, the Association of Herbalists of Mozambique (AERMO), which they have formalized and registered and of which she is national president. In an interview conducted shortly after the coup, Dona Banú, reflecting on the original goals of the organization and the failure to attain them precipitated by these internal politics, said:

> As long as there are people with this kind of greed, AMETRAMO will not move forward, it will not develop. . . . In each plant each [healer] has his/her knowledge. This was the exchange of experience that we came to discuss when we had meetings. But it's not possible . . . because when we're in a meeting, there's that greed for power. . . . It's for this reason that even the Ministry of Health itself . . . keeps us at a distance, it's because of these contradictions that exist amongst us. . . . It's not possible . . . because in the final analysis, these healers are not looking at their careers in terms of being people who cure other people. They only think in terms of contradictions because that guy shouldn't be in charge, and this one can't be ahead of that one, and I too want to be in charge. It can't be this way. . . . It's not possible for everyone to be a *chefe*.

Despite Dona Banú's allusions to a higher purpose for AMETRAMO based on principles of communal goals, shared experience, and a dedication to healing above politics, in practice, political maneuvering and the quest for power and authority are the stuff of AMETRAMO's day-to-day operation. At the provincial and district levels, AMETRAMO Tete's main preoccupation is extracting membership dues and fines for inappropriate behavior from its members. The paying of dues is tied to the officializing of healers' work: in order to practice legally (in AMETRAMO's terms), healers must pay the dues that entitle them to a license and/or official membership documents. AMETRAMO officers imply or claim that this is government policy and that healers who practice without proper payment and documentation are breaking the law, which can result in fines and/or jail time, although AMETRAMO's policies do not actually have the force of law. The population of Tete, long the victims of various kinds of extractive and even violent forces, have been convinced not to question the legitimacy of apparent authorities and their demands. And so they either pay or hide their healing practices from AMETRAMO officials or flee at their approach.

Resistance to AMETRAMO's extractiveness sometimes takes the form of interpretation and rumor (cf. White 2000). Pedro Dos Santos and Manuel Olímpio, both now deceased, were two of the provincial-level leaders of AMETRAMO Tete appointed in 1992. Pedro and Manuel and their colleagues applied themselves to extracting membership fees, dues, and fines from healers throughout the province, part of which they were to send on to Dona Banú at the national headquarters in Maputo, although Dona Banú never received anything. When Pedro and Manuel died of wasting diseases within a year of each other in 2000–2001, many people said it was the result of power struggles among the AMETRAMO leadership, that the various *chefes* had used witchcraft against one another in skirmishes over relative authority and control of funds. But one AMETRAMO leader, an older man who had been involved with the association from the beginning, had another explanation. He said the deaths were the result of the vengeance of the spirit of a particularly powerful healer who was fed up with being forced by the AMETRAMO leaders to pay money that went into their own pockets instead of toward the good of the association.

The political style of AMETRAMO in the provincial capital has reached into the districts in partial and variable ways. The two districts where I did the majority of my research provide examples of the range of AMETRAMO activity. In Angónia, AMETRAMO is strong; in Macanga, it is weak (in inverse relationship, then, to the churches discussed above). The difference reflects, in part, the entrepreneurial ambitions and abilities of particular individuals in their roles as leaders—most notably among them Gabrieli.

As mentioned above, one of Gabrieli's primary concerns as president of AMETRAMO Angónia is witch eradication, a preoccupation and pursuit that has been a part of life throughout this part of Africa for at least 150 years (Chakanza 1985; Richards 1970 [1935]). When I spoke with him in 1998, Gabrieli described for me his recent anti-witch campaign, in which he went from village to village in Angónia "vaccinating"[5] people against witchcraft; he applied anti-witch medicine that caused any of those so treated who were witches to either stop their practices or die. As a part of this campaign, he also sought out and confiscated witchcraft-related materials, including medicines for doing witchcraft against other people and stores of human flesh (the preferred food of witches), which he found buried in people's yards or hidden in their grain bins. In the context of the late 1990s, the president spoke of his work against witches not in terms of religion or morality but in terms of development and service to the government. He showed me a basket filled with small stoppered gourds of various shapes and said:

> See this? These are traditional magical substances which we recovered from the rural area of the district. . . . I have been working with a group [of AMETRAMO members] and we walk together out into the rural areas doing this work. In order to calm those areas. Now, this work that we are doing we are doing also for the development of the country, because we are protecting the lives of people within the population. The government itself doesn't know how magic is done, but it knows that some people are doing strange things. The government is not going to manage to overcome this kind of problem that we are talking about. The ones who have the power to overcome this type of problem are the traditional doctors. . . . Therefore, I would like it very much if the government had more respect for us, the people who are doing this work. Because as it is we are like abandoned people. We do not have the full appreciation of the government. We have been abandoned although we are working day and night for the government.

Gabrieli constructs his (and AMETRAMO's) relationship to the government as one of mediation. Healers mediate between the population and the government, taking up those aspects of governance which the state does not have the knowledge or expertise to accomplish. Although Gabrieli's comments reflect the tensions inherent in the relationship between AMETRAMO and the government, they also reveal his attempt to position healers as necessary to the government, as separate from the general population in what they know and have to offer to the well-being of the nation. As Gabrieli points out, AMETRAMO needs the state, but he also takes pains to show that the state needs AMETRAMO and the knowledge and ability of healers that is contained within the organization.

As president of AMETRAMO, Gabrieli's charge is all the healers of Angónia, which includes not just *aneneri* but also healers who work without spirits or who work with ancestor spirits. However, the vast majority of healing activity taking place in Angónia at the time of my fieldwork was in the hands of the *aneneri,* and Gabrieli also at least partially identified as a *neneri,*[6] so much of AMETRAMO's work under his leadership centered on the prophets and the maintenance of what he deemed to be standards of appropriate behavior for this community. A great concern and recurring topic of discussion for Gabrieli during the time that I knew him was the case of a group of *aneneri* he considered to be transgressors of the dangerous divides between medicine, religion, and politics.

Among his confiscated goods, Gabrieli had a large bundle of prophet clothing, the long gowns, hats, and belts adorned with appliquéd crosses that make up the uniforms specified by the spirits of *aneneri.* He explained that he had uncovered a group of *aneneri* operating in a remote part of the district. According to Gabrieli, the transgressions of these *aneneri* were first, that the leader of this group and his followers claimed to be a "church," an "unregistered" and "unknown" church called "Citizen," organized by Malawians. More seriously, he claimed, this leader was using his church and healing activities to spread propaganda for RENAMO, the opposition political party in Mozambique (although there was little evidence to support this claim). Describing this group, he said:

> At first we didn't realize that the objective of these healers was in terms of secret political activity. These healers were working in two ways, as traditional healers and also politically . . . in favor of RENAMO. They have a church called Citizen. . . . This is a church unknown to the Mozambican government. . . . We were awaiting the [Mozambican] elections, and as Chissano already won, we need to look at this situation again and send this [leader of Citizen] back to his own country or do something else. Because this is unfavorable to and is weakening those traditional healers who are obeying the order of the government. . . . In the registers, Citizen is unknown. It is an illegal church. . . . We have identity cards, we have documents, we have credentials, and we have lists so that we can confirm what [Mozambican] healers are doing. These [Mozambicans who involved themselves with Citizen] were healers, but they changed the situation, they changed the idea. They entered into this church. They pretend that they are traditional healers but they are also members of Citizen.

As with his approach to witchcraft eradication, Gabrieli is putting forward a model of healers and their expertise as crucial to and in sync with the development of the state. But in this case, the boundaries that must be policed fall within the community of healers.

One of the *aneneri* who experienced firsthand Gabrieli's campaign against Citizen was a healer named Yosua. He related his experiences as follows:

> One time I called a meeting of *aneneri* and they came and got me and took me away and I didn't even know what was happening. When they took me, I had to pay money in order to get out of jail. . . . It happened that a few days after the meeting, we were taken by [a fiscal officer of AMETRAMO] . . . and he took us to the police in Domue. When we arrived there they asked the police to hold us for five days. But the police asked, why should we hold these people? What did they do? [The man who had brought us] didn't manage to explain to the police. The police continued to say that they were only going to accept if there was a document which proved that this was true. They showed a document from the Vila [from Gabrieli] and the police accepted to keep us for two days and said that they had to come get us from the jail on Thursday to take us to the Vila to resolve this problem. On Thursday the men came and picked us up from the jail and carried us to the Vila. There in the Vila we didn't go to the police, but went directly to the house of Gabrieli, who is the one who had given the order to arrest us. There at his house he began to threaten us, saying, You are wanted in Maputo, the president of the Republic [Chissano] wants to meet you because you violated laws. Then we said, We're sorry, Mr. Gabrieli, we didn't kill anyone. If we did something wrong, please let's resolve it here and not speak of police and going to Maputo. Then he decided that we ought to pay 4,000 kwacha, each person. And we agreed and the story ended there. . . . He said that if you practice traditional medicine it's not permitted to combine it with prayers or something else, that it's not permitted to combine the two things at the same time.

As the state made traditional medicine its business through attempts to limit or curtail the activities of healers, so healers in the guise of AMETRAMO have taken up the means and methods of the state in order to police their own. And from the perspective of Yosua and other healers, AMETRAMO, in the guise of Gabrieli, *is* the state. This approach does not include the community-building that takes place at the hands of mothers and bishops. Although ostensibly in service of an association, the power of presidents such as Gabrieli derives as much from alienation and exclusion as from connection and inclusion. Although all three varieties of leaders work diligently to erect boundaries, some are more interested in containing people and practices within the boundaries they construct, whereas others are more concerned with what and whom their boundaries keep out.

Conclusion: Constructing Authority

The three leadership and institutional styles described here provide three lenses on the construction of authority in the context of prophet healing in

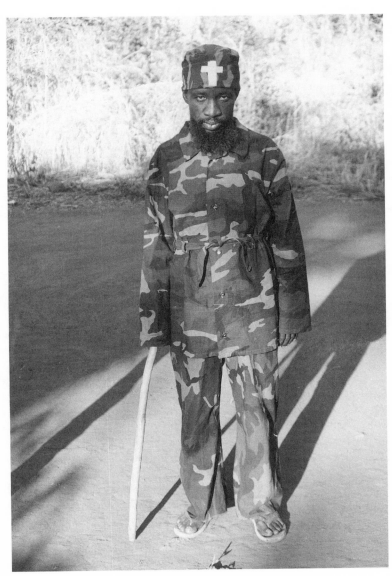
Yobu, a prophet healer and AMETRAMO leader.

northern Tete. The first, exemplified by Magdalena and her followers, is that
which grows from the actual work of *neneri* healing and the mechanisms of the
"cult of affliction." In this model, an individual healer creates authority by
discovering *neneri* spirits in other people, who then become the healer's spiritual "children" and followers. The second model of authority, exemplified by
Yosefe and Citizen Church, is imposed from above and justifies itself through

claims to gendered institutional power based on the spiritual authority of the church. Its historical model is the various Christian churches that have established themselves in the region. The third model is that based in and modeled on the power of the state, as exemplified by Gabrieli and AMETRAMO. In this model, the power structure is also imposed from above. Its authority is justified by the presumed legitimacy of the state, buttressed by its explicit linkings with other organs of the state (for example, the party and the police), and backed up with the trappings of the state in the form of bureaucracy, identification cards, dues or taxes, and so forth. A key difference between the first model, of spiritual mothering, and the second and third, linked to church and state, is that the production of authority through spiritual mothering is relatively transparent. That is, participants and onlookers can see where this power comes from and witness the process of its accumulation. In the second and third models, in contrast, any justification for the processes by which power is assigned, accumulated, and maintained is opaque: participants cannot see why this power is merited, although they can clearly see the ways in which it is enacted.

On the one hand, these healer-leaders and their work reflect the long process of exchange between the spiritual powers of healers and the political forms of church and state. Healing and healers are caught up in the politics of church and state, and they have also caught them and made them their own. If the state has intruded in healing practices, healers have also adopted the bureaucratic style and organization of the state in their own association. If the church has historically impressed its exhortations and prohibitions on the daily lives of the populace, healers have also taken up the narratives, material culture, and organizational style of the church and incorporated them into their own procedures. However, these larger historical and social forces provide only the context in which particular individuals operate. Although the large-scale forces (long-term, regional or national, historical, cultural) are always in evidence, the small-scale, localized, ephemeral forces, the particularities of individual entrepreneurs at any one moment in time, are also profound in their effect. Although they act in a sense as individuals, the power of these entrepreneurs is social. Indeed, there is a blurring of the boundary between the individual leader and the institution he/she leads. Often, healer-leaders traffic in the trappings and rhetoric of institutionalization as much as they produce any concrete evidence of it.

These institutions, their leaders, and the models of power-building they represent are not discrete but are intertwined and overlapping. These intersections reflect the very nature of therapeutic entrepreneurialism, its voracious resourcefulness and constant venturing across limits and boundaries. Indeed, as shown here, these entrepreneurs even pilfer styles, titles, and strategies from one another.[7] Also notable in the work of these entrepreneurs is their ability to make assets of resources of many kinds and scales, both concrete and conceptual, mundane and fantastic, both things themselves and narratives about or replicas of those things. In the hands of these therapeutic entrepreneurs, a government document, a spirit presence, a style of dancing, a Christian symbol sewn on a piece of cloth, a gesture, a threat, a rumor, a memory can all be put to good use, combined to create a new entity, familiar and yet unprecedented enough to be compelling to others. In this sense, these entrepreneurs are consummate politicians, making much out of little, constructing social bodies and their positions of authority within them through complex imaginaries. The work of entrepreneurial individuals to establish themselves as leaders in this setting is performed as a careful political dance among a postcolonial population profoundly suspicious of and ambivalent about power itself. Both the "leaders" and the "followers" in this dance attempt to make sense of and put order to an oftentimes unruly set of experiences. These therapeutic entrepreneurs work hard in a context of "disorder" to establish new orthodoxies of their own construction, drawing on elements from both dominant and subaltern populations of both the past and present. Their success depends on the savvy and creativity of their border work.

Notes

The research upon which this chapter is based would not have been possible without the patience, sensitivity, and insight of my research assistant Pedro Rodrigues. I would also like to thank the many prophets who shared their experiences and practices so generously with me. The paper benefited greatly from comments by Nathalie Arnold, Steven Feierman, Stacey Langwick, Tonya Taylor, Rijk van Dijk, Meghan Vaughan, Richard Werbner, Harry West, and an anonymous reviewer for Indiana University Press. Funding for the project was provided by IIE/Fulbright and the Social Science Research Council.

1.   Scarry (1985) examines the way intense pain, as in torture, dismantles the lifeworld of the sufferer; pain, she suggests, is "world-destroying" in that it systematically reduces the field of consciousness to the body and its immediate environs. Drawing on Scarry, Good suggests that illnesses that entail chronic pain similarly "unmake the world" (1994, 116–134). I use the phrase here to underline the linkage between individual and social bodies in *neneri* experience and practice. Most prophets came to be so through the simultaneous experiences of physical suffering (in the form of illness) and social suffering (in the form of warfare and dislocation). In turn, prophet healing seeks to "remake" individual bodies through healing and social bodies by constructing new moral communities.

2.   The names used in this chapter are spirit names or pseudonyms.

3.   A number of researchers of African history have noted that the reading of the Bible, as introduced by missionaries, has frequently been interpreted by Africans as a powerful ritual act and tool (Comaroff and Comaroff 1991, 192; Hofmeyr 1991, 644; Harries 2001, 418)

4.   In his work on urban South African Zionist churches, Kiernan suggests that leadership within the churches is enacted in the counterpointal partnership between two types, the prophet and the preacher. As he describes it, the volatile, uncontrolled energy of the prophet acts in a fragmenting way on the group, whereas the more ordered, controlled energy of the preacher acts to

consolidate it (Kiernan 1976b; 1990, 359). In a parallel way, he describes Zion-ist rituals as revealing a dialectical relationship between "authority and enthu-siasm" (Kiernan 1976a; 1990, 169–183). Scripture, in this context, is key, he says, because it provides the substance of preaching and is thus the source of the "constitutive" force of the preacher, in contrast to the "centripetal" force of the prophet (Kiernan 1976b, 363). Kiernan describes these contrasting ele-ments as complementary and does not note the gender dynamics involved, whereas I interpret the relationship between preacher and prophet as the site of a gendered struggle between two approaches to power-building.

5. Anti-witchcraft vaccination entails making small cuts in the skin at various points on the body with a razor blade and rubbing in medicinal substances composed of desiccated, pulverized medicinal roots in a base of oil or some other liquid.

6. Gabrieli claimed to have a variety of spirits, including prophet spirits, animal spirits, and other spirits not typically encountered in this region. He was thus able to identify himself with a variety of individuals and communities and to distinguish himself as unique.

7. This process is similar to what Gramsci described regarding the reciprocal assimilation of elites. I am indebted for this insight to Richard Werbner, who suggested this similarity in his comments as discussant for the American An-thropological Association panel at which the paper was first presented in 2002.

3 Of Markets and Medicine: The Changing Significance of Zimbabwean *Muti* in the Age of Intensified Globalization

David Simmons

Crisis, it might be said, is the norm in contemporary Zimbabwe, where the effects of economic structural adjustment, governmental corruption and mismanagement, privatization of health care, landlessness, rapid urbanization, and HIV/AIDS are now embedded in the normal patterns of sociality. This backdrop of constant crisis provides a lens through which to look at how it is that a globalizing economy, shifting flows of information and technology, and new configurations of transnational control and power have provided pathways and routes for African vernacular medicine and its practitioners to transform themselves (see Comaroff and Comaroff 1997). Much of this transformation occurs within and across what were presumed to be discreet boundaries around various forms of healing practices ("traditional" and "modern") and sociospatial positionalities (rural and urban, local and global). Indeed, chronic crises have helped destabilize many of these presumed boundaries and have created spaces for social actors to further destabilize, break down, transcend, and mediate old boundaries or create new ones.

This destabilization of boundaries occurs within the context of downward trends in health outcomes, government services, economic opportunities, and educational prospects in part due to the adoption of an economic structural adjustment program in the early 1990s.[1] The health sector has been particularly hard hit with the introduction of user fees that have amounted to a tenfold increase in charges for consultations, medications, and hospitalizations (Bassett, Bijlmakers, and Sanders 1997). In Harare, for example, basic health care delivery has deteriorated to the point that patients and their relatives often have to provide their own drugs, food, and other basic goods because many government hospitals can no longer provide them due to severe budget cuts. For many poor and middle-class Zimbabweans, translocally produced medicines have been placed completely out of economic reach. This disruption in the availability of health-related goods, services, and products in the formal sector has, in turn, created a health care vacuum that is being filled with African vernacular healing practices and products. Always present, African vernacular medicine has responded—for better and for worse—to this disorder in the formal health care sector in innovative and novel ways.

It is within this field of complicated social action that I focus on a national organization of practitioners of African vernacular medicine, the Zimbabwe National Traditional Healers Association (ZINATHA), and on individual healers. Currently, these self-described "traditional healers" are engaging with new forms of entrepreneurial activity whereby they are attempting to professionalize and commoditize African vernacular medicine while simultaneously maintaining claims to its "authenticity." Understanding the deployment of this maneuver requires us to understand something about the categories of "traditional" medicine and "modern" medicine which they (and others) utilize and invoke: "traditional" and "modern" medicine "do not describe received empirical realities. They are analytic constructs whose heuristic utility depends entirely on the way in which they are deployed to illuminate historically specific phenomena" (Comaroff and Comaroff 1999, 294). Discursive and material activities associated with healing produce these constructs and they shape and constitute a particular version of them, which is used and deployed by different actors for different ends.

In this way, healers are involved in a complicated positioning and repositioning of themselves—their knowledge, their medicines, their alliances—that constitutes the demarcations around categories. Healers in Zimbabwe do not constitute a homogeneous bloc of like-minded practitioners. Healers often operate in contradiction to one another, drawing on a heterogeneity of variable and shifting notions of "science" and "tradition," of "authenticity" and "efficacy," all sources of legitimacy that can, however, undermine one another. Healers draw on the full spectrum of these sources and deploy them for a variety of ends on a variety of scales (from the individual to the group and from the local to the international). A focus on a healing organization and on individual healers helps illustrate the role of healers not only as brokers—mediating the broad scope of these forms of knowledge and experience—but as border guards, policing and controlling the flow of resources in which they work. Healers divide, demarcate, and construct fences around, between, and sometimes through different domains of knowledge, experience, and practice. This chapter is an effort to illustrate this process among Zimbabwean healers.

ZINATHA Enterprises Private Limited

When I visited ZINATHA headquarters one day in 1999, I was surprised to see medicines in carefully labeled bottles on the shelves above the receptionist's desk. "What are these?" I asked one of the office administrators.

"We sell these here now," said Giles, the assistant office manager, handing me a sheet of paper. The paper, it turned out, was a share certificate for the company formed in 1997 which produced and sold the medicine, ZINATHA Enterprises Private Limited (ZEPL). Gordon Chavunduka, president of ZINATHA, writes (1999, 44): "Because of the rising demand for traditional medicine in the society, ZINATHA established a pharmaceutical company in 1997, which was registered as ZINATHA Enterprises Private Limited. The company assists by producing in large quantities those medicines in great demand." The mass production of such medicines by an organization designed to support the practices of *n'anga* greatly interested me. On the one hand, it seemed that such production practices wiped out a very important aspect of the curative process, namely the face-to-face interaction between healer and patient. On the other hand, I wondered if selling mass quantities of *muti* through ZINATHA headquarters would undermine the ability of individual *n'anga* to sell their own individually harvested and processed medicines.[2] Would patients—at least the ones that visited ZINATHA's headquarters—eschew a consultation with a healer if they could just buy their medications over the counter, so to speak? Giles explained that it was individual *n'anga* who indeed benefited from the sale of the medicines; 70 percent of the profit was returned to them (e.g. those responsible for harvesting/processing the medicine), while 30 percent was retained by ZEPL. *N'anga* were welcome to bring in medicinal plants they thought were particularly effective in treating certain afflictions. If they did indeed prove to be effective, ZEPL would then begin processing the medicines for mass consumption. Medicines I saw for sale were usually in powder form, encased in capsules. None of these, to my knowledge, contained artificial preservatives, which would have meant they were no longer "traditional," according to the ZINATHA office administrator (see below). None, to my knowledge, had undergone clinical trials to verify their safety and efficacy.

On a related point, in 1999 ZINATHA asked the government to allocate five large commercial farms under the land redistribution exercise to enable its members to grow medicinal plants. Gordon Chavunduka argued that unless action was taken to meet the increasing demand for medicinal plant use in Zimbabwe, there would likely be a critical shortage of traditional medicines in the next twenty to thirty years—a sentiment similar to the one held by the Global Programme on AIDS and the Traditional Medicine Programme of the WHO (see, e.g., WHO 1989).

As ZINATHA was currently in talks with an unnamed British partner over exporting Zimbabwean *muti* overseas, such speculation may not have been far off the mark. Allegedly, ZINATHA had been approached by the company especially for those medicines that assisted barren couples in conception. Among the particular medicines being considered were those of faith healer Boniface Mponda, whose "holy water" had allegedly already helped thousands of local couples have children. Local newspapers trumpeted the potential partnership, one holding forth in a triumphant tone: "If the partnership is successful, and the Zimbabwean traditional medicine is exported, this could turn out to be a breakthrough in the world of Zimbabwean traditional medicine."[3] As this chapter was being written, nothing had yet come of this partnership.

The School of African Medicine

Another ambitious facet of ZINATHA's attempted professionalization of African therapeutic systems was an effort to build the first school of African medicine in Zimbabwe. Part of the motivation for opening the school, according to Chavunduka, was that the traditional method of teaching apprentices in the field had been disrupted by the new social order. "Traditional healers," he explained in a local newspaper, "used to take about three years teaching an apprentice, but it's no longer possible because most people are now living apart and if it is in town, it's not possible to do an intensive course."[4]

After registering with the Ministry of Higher Education and Technology in December of 1998 and failing to secure funding from the Ministry of Health and Child Welfare, ZINATHA decided to fund the project on its own. The school was to be run like any other medical school, and a syllabus had been drawn up as of July 1999. The program was to be divided into four mutually reinforcing sections: culture and health, religion and health, medicines, and medical practice.

Acknowledging that some Western-educated leaders look down upon the idea of starting a school of African medicine in Zimbabwe, Chavunduka argued that "such people were brainwashed by the type of Western education they received so they look down upon anything that is African."[5] More likely, such alleged critics were casting doubts on the likelihood of the school's success given ZINATHA's ambitious (and sometimes outrageous) projects, many of which have never been completed.

These activities—mass-producing *materia medica*, starting a formal school of African medicine—raise the critical question: When does "traditional" medicine become "Western" medicine? I asked this question of an administrator of ZINATHA. His response:

> Let me start by highlighting a point: more than 70 percent of drugs available today come from plants. That is, medicinal plants. And when we speak of medicinal plants, we are speaking of traditional medicine. But these processes of extraction, processing, and production . . . these would lead us to calling them "Western" medicine. Coming back to your question, when medicine has gone past the stage of being dispensed in a calabash (*gona*), of being dispensed in the form of bark, leaf, and root form, and so forth, and it is mixed with preservatives for ensuring shelf life . . . surely, when you mix it with chemicals, like preservatives, etc., it ceases to be traditional medicine.

And yet ZINATHA had been involved in training healers in just such practices—making medicines available in capsule form, bottled and clearly labeled for consumption, since 1988. Such training was and is an attempt to "professionalize"—read "modernize"—traditional medicine (see Last and Chavunduka 1986), the belief being that medicine stored in calabashes was unhygienic and that healers were more prone to prescribe incorrect dosages.[6] Healers still usually dispense herbal medicines wrapped in newspaper on which is written the dosage, and they also give dosage instructions verbally. Of the 100 healers that I interviewed over the course of five years (1995–1999), the vast majority continued to store their *materia medica* in calabashes, distributing medicine in this way.

Motives for changing the way healers collect, process, and store medicines may be taken at face value. From the perspective of ZINATHA administrators, such efforts are an attempt to better regulate this process and offer a more hygienic, superior product to clients. On the other hand, the deployment of the trope of "professionalization" (as used by ZINATHA's leadership) destabilizes the boundary around what has historically been seen as an "unprofessional" profession: traditional healing. Professionalization, as a process and end product, lends local healing an air of formal authority and businesslike standards that, historically, healers have been accused of lacking. The deliberate transgression of this divide (professional/unprofessional) signals ZINATHA's attempts to refashion its perception in the public's eye, particularly as consumers of health services and products demand more "professional" standards.

Shona Medicines

As much as professionalization can be seen as updating and "modernizing" the production of local medicine, it is also important to remember that *muti,* as an analytical category, has always enjoyed a certain transgressive quality in how it is defined. In the context of Shona society, the term "medicine" assumes a much more elastic meaning than Western understandings of the term. For Westerners, the term signifies any preventive and/or curative substance, and this is certainly true in Shona society as well. Additionally, however, medicine also refers to metaphysical power that may be protective or, alternately, dangerous or punitive.

Medicines, or *muti,* in their curative and metaphysical embodiments figure prominently in the lives of Shona peoples. From life's nascent beginnings during conception to life's final passage into death—and a new life among the ancestors—*muti* is an important mediating presence. When a child is born, for example, there is great concern about the anterior fontanel of the infant as this is regarded as the weakest part of the body, where sickness or poison can enter. Any disturbance in the fontanel is called *chipande* or *nhova.* Treatment typically requires a poultice of a tarry, thick mixture that is applied over the fontanel. Likewise, various roots soaked in water are used to bathe babies in as a way of fortifying their systems and protecting them from illness (Chavunduka 1978; Gelfand 1964).

As a child matures into an adult, various afflictions are visited upon him or her, all of which require recourse to *muti* in its metaphysical and curative manifestations. And because these afflictions may be caused by antisocial acts, such as upsetting or angering ancestral spirits (*vadzimu*) or a witch (*muroyi*) or failure to perform certain ritual practices or taboos (Gelfand, Mavi, Drummond, and Ndemera 1985; Chavunduka 1980; Bourdillon 1998), *muti* assumes a very personal role and is associated with an individual's identity; it signifies ideas of personal power and agency, the ability to protect oneself and others, to cure or to harm and kill one's enemies if necessary (cf. Bierlich 1999; Comaroff and Comaroff 1997). Crawford (1967, 103) explains: "Medicines are used to protect one against witchcraft; to pass examinations; to win the love of an unwilling woman; to see in the dark; to grow crops successfully; to dispel the *ngozi* and to raise it; to create or cure a witch; and for many other purposes."

A review of these diverse uses helps underline the fact that the felt need for medicines in Zimbabwe is very great. Nationwide, 10 percent of children die before their fifth birthday—mostly from very treatable afflictions such as malaria and diarrheal diseases. In certain locations, the infant/child mortality rate appears to be rising (UNICEF 1994). In the context of extreme poverty and lack of access to even basic health care, the diarrhea, coughs, and fevers that families are medicating are potentially deadly. Parasites, anemia, diarrhea, tuberculosis, and HIV and other sexually transmitted diseases are common. No doubt the incidence of health problems could be reduced by improving economic conditions and public health care measures, but barring such improvements people are sick and want curative care in the form of medicines. In such a context of high mortality and morbidity from infectious diseases, medicines are of crucial value for ordinary people and health professionals alike (Whyte and Birungi 2000, 131).

Added to this high disease burden is the decline and disarray of government health services. The lack of pay increases and benefits under economic structural adjustment has hastened the outward flight of Zimbabwean-trained doctors and nurses both from government service and from Zimbabwe. The number of nurses per capita fell by 17 percent between 1988 and 1993 (Loewenson and Chisvo 1994). This, in turn, has had an adverse effect on health services in the public sector. Enforcement of fee collection combined with an apparent deterioration in the staffing situation and quality of service at these facilities appears to be causing profound and negative changes in health-seeking behavior, especially for mothers and children. The observed overall decline in 1992 in the outpatient attendance rate among children under five years of age as compared to the same period in 1988–1991, for example, may reflect an increasing reluctance on the part of mothers to take their children to health care facilities because of fees and tends to confirm Hongoro and Chandiwana's (1994) study on the impact of fee collection on delivery of health care services.

One effect of this crisis in governmental health services—as symbolized by ongoing strikes by doctors and nurses—was the media's finger-pointing at *n'anga* as "cashing in" on the crisis. The March/April 1997 issue of *Catholic News* proclaimed, "ZINATHA Cashes in on Nurses' and Junior Doctors' Strike, Mission Nurses Not Involved." In a subtitle, the article painted the motives of *n'anga* as less than noble: "Local *n'angas* cashed in on last year's critical strike by government medical workers around the country, making huge turnovers from the desperate and ill." The article went on to say that ZINATHA "seized the opportunity to maximize its earnings by opening its magic doors to the many poor people who could not afford the high fees of private doctors and hospitals." The administration manager for ZINATHA at the time, Boniface Makoni, is quoted as saying: "The strike brought about two faces. Firstly, many poor people who could not afford the huge fees of private hospitals turned to us for treatment. So we had a very big turnover at the peak of the strike. Secondly, we were faced with emergency cases we could not deal with, such as fractured bones. We referred such cases to conventional hospitals, but only the lucky few got treatment, and there was nothing we could do to help out the situation." He wisely went on to say that although the strike brought in "huge earnings" for ZINATHA, money was not the first priority for *n'anga*. "We value most the life of the patient, not the money that we make out of him."

This chronic malaise within the formal health care system has helped create a void that is quickly being filled with new and hybrid forms of therapeutic practice and *muti*. For example, from a curative standpoint, *muti* refers to various locally produced and commercially available herbs—usually available in the wild or at local markets, where some are even carefully labeled and bottled for sale[7]—as well as Western pharmaceuticals, usually in the form of capsules and pills. And very often this distinction may be blurred as some medicine sellers may package locally produced/grown herbs in used, or recycled, translocally produced medicine bottles. Additionally, some sellers give their herbal concoctions biomedical-sounding names such as "A.C.T.5," "Profferon," and "GK17," perhaps with the hope that buyers will view these medicines as more effective than those which are called by their local, and more common, names.[8]

Medicine within Zimbabwe signifies ritual curative substances and practices as well. Material curative substances—medicinal plants encapsulated, bottled, and labeled for sale—are much more apt to be called "Western" than their ritual counterparts. Divination through the throwing of bones or through spirit possession, for example, is less likely to be labeled "Western." However, this, too, is changing.

In its metaphysical dispensation, *muti* may refer to "protective" medicines, such as substances and materials in the form of talismans or charms, which either through ingestion or external application protect the client from diseases, evil spirits or bad luck (*mamhepo*), or enemies. It may also refer to harmful or punitive medicines used, for example, to punish a spouse's alleged lovers,[9] to hurt an enemy, or to gain someone else's property. Love potions also fall under the rubric of supernatural medicines. Other medicines, such as *mangoromera*, are used to instill moral qualities such as courage and strength (see Gelfand 1964). You would not find these medicines in capsule form, neatly bottled and labeled at ZINATHA headquarters.

The use of medicinal plants—and occasionally in conjunction with animal, and sometimes human, parts—for curative purposes is quite common. Medicines are infused with their curative capabilities usually through sacrifice and/or the pouring of libations in conjunction with prayers. Thus, *muti*'s potency is not self-evident; that is, it comes from external sources—the ancestors or healing spirits—and is given agentive power through men and women's intentions. The ability to give *muti* and to use it, to act as a curative agent, implies a moral relationship with the ancestors, healing spirits, and/or God, without whose support the *muti* remains inert.[10] Curative practice, in this sense, is the site par excellence of mediation between the human and the divine.[11]

This relationship underscores the fact that healing is a gift bestowed by these various agents and that malpractice can result in the gift being taken away.[12] A corollary is that a medicine's efficacy—that is, its ability to work—is contingent on the careful maintenance of these connections. A healer whose *muti* gains a reputation for not working is suspected not only of being a charlatan but of upsetting the careful balance of these relationships.

On occasion, the ancestral and/or healing spirits may work to ferret out such individuals, usually in public settings. During a ZINATHA-sponsored workshop in 1996, for example, some spirit mediums became possessed during the playing of traditional music, led by the *mbira,* or thumb piano. One of the spirit-possessed mediums pointed out that several *n'anga* were "fakes." Ritually brewed beer was poured on the back of a goat. When the goat shook the beer from its back, it meant that the meeting could continue with the blessing of the spirits. However, the goat didn't shake the beer from its back and the spirit asked a particular *n'anga* to step to the side. He stepped aside, and the goat shook the beer off. This confirmed the fact that he was indeed a "fake."

Such accusations have become increasingly common both among *n'anga* themselves and between the wider society and *n'anga.* In part, this stems from the perception that more individuals are entering the healing profession as a way to make money.[13] This process may be facilitated by the fact that the Traditional Medical Practitioner's Council and ZINATHA have not yet set a maximum and minimum scale of fees for registered *n'anga* and really do not have the institutional or human resources to enforce such a fee scale even if they had one. Both parties recognize the slipperiness of this issue, particularly with regard to historical arrangements regarding fees. For example, in many rural areas healers do not charge very much—or sometimes anything—for their services, viewing their practice not as a business but as a form of community service. Such healers and their families enjoy the reward of high status that comes from their practice and their favored access to the spirit world. In such cases, *n'anga* view fees as tributes to the spirits and not as material reward for themselves. In other cases, *n'anga* who do not receive any fees may expect a patient to give them gifts from time to time when he or she is fully recovered. This payment scenario can become quite expensive.[14]

The lack of a fee structure and lack of an adequate infrastructure to enforce it has resulted in exceptional and widely publicized abuses. Perhaps one of the better-known cases is that of Benjamin Burombo, a Kuwadzana-based herbalist–spirit medium who rose to national fame in 1993 for claiming to have a cure for AIDS. The dreadlocked, self-proclaimed healer of AIDS was known to travel in lavish style with well-dressed body guards and an ostentatious BMW, usually escorted by two Mercedes Benzes. His flamboyant and profligate lifestyle initially made him a media star because journalists at the time, intent on getting the scoop on healers who claimed they could cure the disease, regularly hunted such *n'anga*. Indeed, media frenzy—and the marketing and clientele it helped generate—helps spur the entry of unscrupulous healers into the profession.

As media coverage of Burombo escalated, AIDS patients began filling his Kuwadzana home. He boldly asked his clients to first produce a certificate verifying their HIV-positive status before he treated them. Following a treatment of herbs, and in some cases water,[15] Burombo would advise his patients to go for another HIV test. He claimed that most of these patients returned having been clinically proven to be HIV negative. His patients were usually reluctant to talk about their conditions after undergoing his treatment. Those who did talk had mixed feelings; some said they felt much healthier, others were not so sure.[16] He dismissed as foolish the idea that he submit his *muti* for clinical trials in Europe, arguing that such a scenario where his medicines were processed overseas would result in most patients failing to access the medicines because of costs—something the average Zimbabwean couldn't do anyway under his pricing scheme. He felt that the processing and manufacturing of drugs should remain local so they could be more adequately controlled.

At the height of his fame in 1993, Burombo charged Z$5,000 for a single treatment, roughly the equivalent of what the average worker at the time would earn in one year. Today, in 2004, he has lowered his treatment fee to Z$2,000, arguing that most people cannot afford the higher fees at the moment because of current economic hardships.[17]

Sadly, of course, the price of such treatments is fueled by profound desperation as more and more people living with AIDS seek miracle cures. Aware that such abuses might occur, ZINATHA has regularly admonished healers through various branch and regional meetings for claiming to have a cure for the disease. Likewise, through workshops sponsored by the National AIDS Co-ordination Programme, healers were given a protocol whereby all drugs were to be subjected for clinical trials to evaluate their effectiveness. The Ministry of Health and Child Welfare (MOHCW), through locally based Blair Research, would provide the project funds and employ a full-time researcher to collect data and compile the project report. The MOHCW would also provide patients whose HIV-positive status was confirmed; the patients would be tested at three- and six-month intervals after commencing treatment. ZINATHA would provide a register of traditional healers participating in the project. Unfortunately, the collection and testing of medicinal plants has been inconsistent, and the project was suspended after just a short time. The reasons why are much debated. However, local AIDS activist and counselor Lynde Francis, who participated in Blair Research's clinical trials with *n'anga* said:

> They've never published them [the results] . . . because they proved that [traditional medicine] works. I think they supported those trials because they thought it would prove once and for all that traditional healers were a bunch of charlatans and that it didn't have any effect. And when the trials clearly began to go the other way, I think they backed off because they ran out of funds and they couldn't complete . . . and they didn't analyze the data. They said the data was flawed. They did

publish some preliminary data and it was good, it was really good. It really showed a difference that people were getting higher CD4 counts; better full blood counts, gaining weight. In the year that it ran, they had only, like, 4 deaths out of something like 150 people. It was very very few. And these were people who were coming from the main hospitals [as] outpatients. They were really ill, people with CD4s of 14 and 13, you know. And yet they were not dying. And that alone I thought they would really want to trumpet from the rooftops, but no, they have never really published it. They've never really made much of it at all.

I asked Lynde about the apparent antipathy between the government and n'anga. She explained:

I think it's very difficult to say. . . . A lot of it has to do with the fact that most of the top people in the government were Catholic-educated. They're the product of mission schools. They were taught that traditional healing was witchcraft and to undervalue it. But I still don't think that explains it enough. In this day, they should be aware of it. You know there's more to things than just Western practices. They should have a much more open mind to their own tradition and culture. So I can't say that that's the whole answer, but it's obviously part of the answer.

With limited material and human resources, it seemed to me that the government should have been more interested in at least exploring the role of n'anga in helping combat the spread of HIV/AIDS. Lynde continued:

I don't know the answer to that question. It's something that frazzles and puzzles me tremendously. Why there's this resistance, why there's no real effort to investigate more. ZINATHA is doing stuff on its own, but it's not getting government support for it.

The government, of course, is comprised of people with multiple interests, voices, and opinions, and, in all fairness, there are some in government who are supportive of traditional medicine. Dzivarasekwa member of parliament Edson Wadyehwata, for example, has championed local approaches to combating HIV/AIDS. In particular, he has argued that government should support research into AIDS by traditional healers and desist from "relying on foreigners, otherwise we will be given wrong medication that may kill us faster than AIDS." Wadyehwata has argued that traditional healers have made considerable progress in their research into HIV/AIDS and that they could do more with government support and assistance. Sounding much like Gordon Chavunduka, president of ZINATHA, Wadyehwata has said, "We can't rely on foreign medicine, we need to pursue the traditional Zimbabwean way of researching on medicine otherwise we will be given the wrong medication. . . . We hope government will see what further steps it can take."[18] The question is, of course, Who in government is listening to MP Wadyehwata and what real power does he have in translating his concern into an actionable plan?

These discussions shed light on some of the forces that both motivate and constrain the efforts of n'anga to professionalize and combat diseases such as HIV/AIDS. First, there is the felt need to develop a set fee schedule for healers so that abuses of patients do not occur, abuses which may be more likely in the desperation wrought by HIV/AIDS. Moreover, any apparent abuse on the part of *n'anga* quickly finds its way into print, often perpetuating the public perception that *n'anga* are charlatans just trying to make a quick dollar at the expense of their patients. But ZINATHA does not have the human resources to enforce and monitor fee schedules even in the event that they could get their constituency to agree to them. And given the diverse economic fortunes of their clients, rural *n'anga*, for example, would find it difficult to charge the same fees as their urban counterparts.

Second, external pressures also contribute to the felt need of *n'anga* to professionalize. As medicine becomes increasingly commercialized and mass produced, the clients of *n'anga* may begin to expect local *muti* to follow similar trends; that is, they may expect it to come in labeled bottles in capsule form. As one person living with HIV/AIDS, Tichafa, stated when interviewed about treatment options:

> I'd rather be with the Western people with regard to health. There's no checklist with traditional healers. You can even overdose. I've lost lots of money through these people [traditional healers]. They charge you lots of money for things not proven. The Western way is better—good vitamins and good diet. I had TB once and went down to 47 kilograms. Vitamins and good diet saved me and constant visits to doctors. When you have diarrhea, you don't go to a faith healer for herbs! Right now I'm on a triple combination therapy of DDI, Crixovan, and Zerid.

Responses to such criticism include bottling and labeling medical concoctions and giving them biomedical-sounding names. But while bottling and encapsulating medicines into pill form might seem like a positive move toward professionalization, there is still no testing mechanism in place that would indicate to *n'anga* the level of concentration of active ingredients in such medicines. Patients may have an idea of how much medicine they're getting in bulk form but have no idea of how much they're getting in terms of levels of active ingredients.

The resulting ambiguity of such processes was captured in the popularity of an imported herbal palliative known as Mocrea. At the time, Mocrea was being imported by a local "practitioner of natural medicine," a man who called himself "Dr." Ngwenya, a retired high-ranking military official. During his work with Chinese businesspeople, he came across an herbal palliative called Mocrea (or Tai-Sheng) that was alleged to boost the immune system and was used in China with hepatitis and suppressed immune systems. Ngwenya began importing Mocrea to Zimbabwe, at first approaching Minister of Health and Child Welfare Timothy Stamps to okay the herbal palliative for clinical trials. When Dr. Stamps's okay was not forthcoming, Ngwenya approached then Deputy Minister Tsungirirayi Hungwe, asking her for a couple of AIDS patients on which to prove Mocrea's efficacy. She provided someone who worked at the ministry and one of her cousins. After several weeks' treatment, both, allegedly, were much improved, regaining lost weight and returning to their jobs full-time. After seeing what appeared to be miraculous recoveries, Deputy Minister Hungwe appeared on a national television show in 1996 proclaiming that Mocrea appeared to treat (and reverse) many AIDS-related symptoms (weight loss, loss of appetite, chronic fatigue, etc.).[19] Her television appearance was a marketing coup for Mocrea; HIV/AIDS sufferers and their families and friends began asking about and aggressively seeking it.

Because Mocrea is an herbal palliative (in other words, a medicinal plant), which in the case of Zimbabwe usually falls under the jurisdiction of *n'anga*, Ngwenya filled out an application of certification at ZINATHA and became registered as a "traditional healer" (an herbalist). As such, he had the legal right (in theory) to dispense medicinal plants and herbal palliatives, which he did/does from his clinic. He also gave complimentary boxes of Mocrea to ZINATHA's downtown headquarters for sale—and he continues to do so—as a goodwill token of his certification and registration. In 1996, a 30-capsule bottle cost Z$200 (at the time US$1 equaled Z$7), almost half the monthly income of the average worker at the time. The average bottle, with a recommended dosage of one capsule taken three times a day (more for full-blown AIDS sufferers), lasted ten days.

During my daily visits to ZINATHA headquarters in 1996, I usually encountered several people who were asking about and/or buying Mocrea; the administration manager and his assistant offered advice about dosage. I asked a prominent *n'anga* and ZINATHA executive board member from Epworth about Mocrea and whether or not he prescribed it to his patients. "I don't use it because it has not been tested," he responded. "Healing is a gift from God—not for profit-making. I treat patients who cannot pay. There are negative side effects to Mocrea, for example, getting fat," he continued. He went on to say that people should not go on television extolling the benefits of an untested herb.

The case of Dr. Ngwenya illustrates the general popular ambivalence that ZINATHA exacerbates when it draws from and combines therapeutic resources that are thought to be incompatible. ZINATHA's power in cities such as Harare and Bulawayo, of course, derives precisely from such maneuvers, where it serves a clientele of urban Zimbabweans whose access to both "traditional" and "modern" therapeutic resources is limited. For ZINATHA, such maneuvering is a principle of practice. At the same time, their strength is also their weakness, for to the extent that healers traffic in "modern" medicine, their patients/clients may suspect them of being second-rate practitioners of "traditional" medicine, and to the extent that they practice "traditional" medicine, their patients may suspect them of not keeping up with the times.

Moreover, granting people such as Ngwenya the status of a registered healer creates dissonance within ZINATHA and leads the public to believe that such status can be easily bought, further undermining trust in the practice of healers. According to the Traditional Medical Council, any person who wishes to register as a traditional healer must apply to the registrar and submit an application. Chavunduka (1998, 49) writes that "after submission, all applications are referred to the Council which has the authority to grant registration, if satisfied that the applicant possesses sufficient skill and ability to practice as a traditional medical practitioner and is of good character." Healers who want to register are usually accompanied to the corporate headquarters of ZINATHA by a senior healer who vouches for their training and character. A ZINATHA administrator admitted to me off-handedly that most people "do not refer to Ngwenya as a *n'anga* [but] as that 'Mocrea' guy."

From the perspective of ZINATHA, Ngwenya is appealing because he has high visibility in Harare, he is well spoken, and he is a natural at self-promotion—all traits that are useful to an organization that sees itself as struggling to prove its relevance in a rapidly changing world. However, Ngwenya's involvement in ZINATHA and his efforts to market Mocrea can pose challenges for other *n'anga* and their patients. For *n'anga* it can mean more time, energy, and money spent on "packaging" medicines—just as Mocrea is packaged—that they previously made available in their crude form. Such a process could also mean closer scrutiny by the Zimbabwean Research Council, which typically handles clinical trials of "Western" medicines being introduced to the local market. For some *n'anga,* this could mean the loss of some autonomy in their healing practice. At the same time, *n'anga* are legally prohibited—in theory—from dispensing "Western" medicines; this includes everything from antibiotics to aspirin. If *n'anga* begin processing their medicines in such a way that they are indistinguishable from their Western counterparts, what will that mean in legal terms? For patients, apart from the danger of toxicity mentioned above, there is the question of choice in health care options. If patients feel that the curative practices of *n'anga* are becoming more closely aligned with that of biomedical doctors, they may feel less inclined to visit them, especially for *materia medica.*

Related to this effort at professionalization are the very real constraints placed on *n'anga* by government and the local medical establishment in their efforts to combat diseases such as HIV/AIDS. Whereas historically the government has practiced a policy of benign neglect with regard to the curative practices of *n'anga* in relation to their patients, the HIV/AIDS pandemic has meant increased scrutiny of *n'anga.* Before making public claims about the efficacy of their medicines in treating HIV/AIDS, *n'anga* are required to submit their medicines to government clinical trials. Certainly such scrutiny is justified in a public health emergency, but given the inherent tension between the government, health professionals, and *n'anga,* such scrutiny has the effect of pushing such claims and practices underground. It also reinforces the idea many *n'anga* have that both the government and doctors are interested in monitoring their curative practices only as a way of stealing this knowledge and enriching themselves.

The examples presented here help illustrate the complex positioning and re-positioning of healers that allows them to simultaneously cross, construct, deconstruct, and police boundaries around different domains of knowledge and experience. Certainly such boundary maintenance has been facilitated by the commoditization of indigenous medicine, suspended as it is in a saturating cultural context of capitalism. As with other commodities, market forces shape the value attached to local *muti.* This is increasingly the case as translocal actors and organizations—scientists, researchers, and multinational pharmaceutical organizations—become more interested in African vernacular medicines. These processes of commoditization seem to have accelerated with the continued spread of HIV/AIDS as local and translocal actors search for a "magic bullet." And the epidemic seems to fuel a growing body of unscrupulous healers (and nonhealers) bent on turning a quick profit for themselves or for their clients.

Importantly, however, this process has also been facilitated by the self-conscious positioning of healers as part of the struggle for legal and, perhaps more widely, societal recognition in postcolonial Zimbabwe. For better or for worse, "professionalization" is often seen as "modern," as in the production of capsules in neatly labeled bottles, keeping carefully written notes on patients, and having the proper registration certificates from ZINATHA. As they attempt to balance the demands of a market-driven economy with the demands of the ancestors and healing spirits, healers are placed at a critical crossroads. In this way, "modernity" poses new sorts of possibilities and constraints to Zimbabwean *n'anga*.

On another level, the changing meanings and forms given to medicines in their crude and symbolic forms speaks to healers' and patients' felt interior experiences and their positions in fields of relational power (see Das, Kleinman, Ramphele, and Reynolds 2000). For Zimbabwean healers and the organization that purports to represent them, these changing meanings emerge from the tension of concealing and revealing that is very much embedded in different modes of transgressing and maintaining boundaries. For ZINATHA, this has meant creating a "third way" (to use Bertrand Aristide's term), a neotraditional positionality that is both betwixt and between "traditional" and "modern" healing styles. However, ZINATHA's focus on professionalization—which favors the material packaging of the medicine at the expense of the social/ritual/symbolic relations through which "traditional" medicine is dispensed—makes it vulnerable to being eliminated from the equation altogether and revealing to its clients its marginal position in the modern world.

Drawing on "modern" techniques and practices to enhance their healing repertoires constitutes a high-risk game for ZINATHA healers. Consequently, tracing and retracing boundaries around domains of knowledge and experience has become the principle of practice. Their efforts to simultaneously reify the constructs of "traditional" and "modern" medicine as discreet spheres of knowledge and practice while also drawing from both to create a form of medicine that is "neotraditional" offer the promise of reconciling two systems of knowledge and practice that have historically been thought of as incompatible and antithetical. Time will tell how successful they will be.

Notes

1. As in other parts of Africa, the agreement included austerity measures such as reduction of the budget deficit through decreases in public enterprise

deficits and rationalization of public sector employment; trade liberalization, including price decontrol and deregulation of foreign trade, investment, and production; phased removal of subsidies; devaluation of the local currency; and enforcement and introduction of cost recovery in the health and education sectors.

2. *Muti* are curative substances usually produced by traditional healers, but the term can also refer to Western-produced pharmaceuticals. Whyte and Birungi (2000, 145), in their work in Uganda, note that "African medicines" are not mass produced and marketed on a large scale because local communities are self-sufficient in "traditional medicines."

3. Muponda had been only recently acquitted of sixteen charges of sodomy and four charges of indecent assault. In 1999, Muponda was beginning the long process of rebuilding his practice after the charges. Prior to the charges, he had begun ambitious plans for a hospital in the high-density suburb of Norton. After his criminal charges were made public, many of his donors backed out of the deal.

4. "Traditional Medicines to be Exported," *Zimbabwean Standard*, June 13–19, 1999.

5. Ibid.

6. Deducing the correct dosage is usually the result of years of transmitted oral knowledge. One healer, an herbalist/spirit medium, told me that *n'anga* will usually dream of a particular herb/medicinal plant and even dream its correct use. These dreams, he said, are in part the result of observing animals—monkeys and baboons—in the bush utilizing medicinal plants.

7. Since 1988, ZINATHA has encouraged *n'anga* to bottle their *muti* in an effort to make it more hygienic. It is important to point out that many of the medicine sellers at the markets are not *n'anga*, per se.

8. In a related discussion of medicine use in Uganda, Whyte and Birungi (2000) note that foreign medicines—whether African or non-African—have always held a certain attraction.

9. This is usually the case if a man suspects his wife is committing adultery (I have not come across an equivalent situation for a wife whose husband is committing adultery). The husband will consult a *n'anga* for the proper *muti*, which he will place secretly in her bed or food. Thereafter, any man (other than the husband) that has sexual intercourse with her will contract an affliction known locally as *runyoka*. *Runyoka* is also the name of the *muti*. Symptoms of *runyoka* include fatigue, drastic weight loss, and wasting. If left untreated by a traditional healer, it is said to result in death. As Gelfand and others (1985, 37) point out, there are many types of *runyoka*, the most common being *runyoka rwemago, runyoka rwehamba*, and *runyoka rwemba*. All of these types of *muti* utilize different animal/insect parts (wasps, poisonous snakes, genitals of male and female dogs) which, through sympathetic application, are said to affect the wife's lovers in like manner.

10. See Bierlich 1999; Fortes 1987; Gelfand, Mavi, Drummond, and Ndemera 1985.

11. See Comaroff and Comaroff 1997, 333.

12. Chavunduka (1998, 44) points out that in the case of spirit mediums, it is strongly believed that ancestors and healing spirits can withdraw the healing skill bestowed upon the individual if it is offended.

13. See, for example, "Act Against AIDS Cure Charlatans—Nyazema," (Zimbabwe) *Herald,* July 23 1996; "Bogus Healer Fined," (Zimbabwe) *Daily News,* June 17, 1999; "False Prophets Swindle Thousands of Dollars," (Zimbabwe) *Daily News,* May 12, 1999.

14. Chavunduka 1999.

15. AIDS counselor Lynde Francis and her husband, a popular Zimbabwean musician who eventually died of AIDS-related complications, visited Burombo and received just such a treatment of water.

16. Tichafa, also quoted in this chapter, also visited Burombo. He was openly suspicious of Burombo's treatment regimen.

17. This is still considered exorbitant where, in 1999, the average worker made about Z$1,500 per month.

18. "Measures Urged to Protect Aids Orphans," *Zimbabwe Daily News,* May 13, 1999.

19. Her appearance on national television and her acceptance of Mocrea provided a great deal of grist for the media mill and further ammunition for discrediting Minister Stamps. Comment in the June 24, 1996, *Zimbabwe Herald* proclaimed: "One day Stamps was publicly denouncing Mocrea and all other conventional medicines whose inventors have claimed they can cure AIDS and the next day his deputy, Cde. Tsungirirayi Hungwe, was relaying on television personal experiences of a relative whose AIDS symptoms had been reversed by the intake of the Chinese concoction."

4 Money, Modernity, and Morality: Traditional Healing and the Expansion of the Holy Spirit in Mozambique

James Pfeiffer

The extraordinary expansion of Pentecostals and African Independent Churches (AICs) influenced by Pentecostalism over the last decade in central Mozambique marks a dramatic shift away from reliance on "traditional" healers, known as *nyanga* or *n'anga* in Shona dialects or *curandeiros* in Portuguese, to treat persistent afflictions believed to have spiritual causes. The AICs, which include Zionist and Apostolic movements with roots in South Africa and Zimbabwe, and more mainstream Pentecostals including various manifestations of the Assemblies of God and the Apostolic Faith Mission, have found fertile ground for growth among the poor in Mozambique, who are recruited primarily through healing.[1] As reported in other areas of Africa, these movements have provoked significant conflict with local *curandeiros;* this conflict is essential to the way that church healers distinguish themselves from traditional practitioners. While demonization of traditional healers by AICs and Pentecostals is widely reported in Africa, there is little in the current literature that explains why this demonization resonates so strongly and attracts so many of the poor or why local healers should lose their legitimacy and perceived efficacy in treating the same illness-causing spiritual afflictions and occult threats that church prophet healers also address.

The success of the movements in southern Africa has been attributed by some to the ways that church healing processes may soothe the trauma of social dislocation, dispersion, and anomie in the transition to urban modernity (see Sundkler 1961; Daneel 1970, 1988, 1992; Oosthuizen 1989, 1992; Bourdillon 1991; Kiernan 1977; Dube 1989). Earlier versions of this approach focused on syncretic healing practices that were thought to provide a bridge back to tradition for disoriented and nostalgic urban migrants presumably bewildered by their new circumstances. In Mozambique, the explanatory models of churches for illness incorporate many of the same local Shona idioms of social distress deployed by traditional healers; however, pastors and prophets have imported the Pentecostal notion of the universal Holy Spirit (Mwiya Mutsene in Chiteve, and Espirito Santo in Portuguese) to provide broad protection, free of charge, against frequent threats from the occult to health and well-being.

Others have debated whether AICs constitute resistance or acquiescence to colonialism and the political economy of apartheid (Ranger 1986; Thomas 1994; Walshe 1991; Schoffeleers 1991; Comaroff 1985). However, given their growing vitality in the post-apartheid period, a new paradigm of sorts has emerged that locates AIC and Pentecostal success within the problematic of globalization and the transition to modernity by emphasizing the churches' rejection of "tradition" in their effort to "break with the past," Pentecostalism's embrace of modernity, and church members' participation in a new social identity that transcends ethnicity and nation (see Corten and Marshall-Fratani 2001; Meyer 1998; Poewe 1994; van der Veer 1996; Coleman 2000; van Dijk 1998). To join these movements, members may also break with their own pasts as represented by ties to family and tradition in rural areas to create new, modern, urban, more individual identities freed from the constraints of rural family demands and "backward" beliefs (Meyer 1998). Traditional healers are vilified and demonized by AICs and Pentecostal movements specifically because they are representative of "tradition" and their healing idioms keep individuals mired in backwardness and poverty, impeding progress toward modernity and prosperity (see Meyer 1993).

However, the illness narratives from the central Mozambican city of Chimoio, which focus on patterns of health-seeking among lay members that precede and motivate the resort to prophet healers, provide conversion stories that do not fit easily within the new paradigm. In these narratives, church members speak less of rejecting the past than of their disillusionment with the intensified commodification of traditional healing in a changing social environment of sharpening income disparities and declining social security—an environment generated in part by economic liberalization and structural adjustment over the last decade. Certainly the many years of war in the post-independence period provoked mass dislocation, shattering local communities and disrupting relationships of social support. While the war was a critical factor in shaping contemporary Mozambique, respondents in the interviews gathered here speak less of the trauma of war and instead emphasize current social circumstances and disruptions.

In this new environment, traditional healing practices have increasingly been tailored and sold to men who often pay high fees to practice, or protect against, sorcery related to obtaining employment or undermining competitors. The market has grown for these kinds of *curandeiro* services as men struggle to obtain scarce jobs in the city amid the lure of potential wealth in the growing economy and *curandeiro* treatments for maternal and child health care have been priced out of range for many women. However, the inflation of fees has had other, perhaps more important, effects on treatment choice. Rising fees in the context of increasingly stark social inequalities taint the legitimacy of the therapeutic processes of *curandeiros* and introduce a skepticism into patient-healer interactions that questions the motives and character of healers. Many *curandeiros* are perceived to be complicit in advancing their clients' fortunes at the expense of others, all while profiting themselves. Remuneration for traditional healing is certainly not new; many *curandeiros* have reportedly received compensation in some form for years in Mozambique. But in the new environment where the social gradient has steepened so quickly, the increasing importance of money to survival and inflation of treatment fees have shifted the market toward those who can pay and have changed the meaning of payment transaction itself in ways that cast doubt on healers' ambitions.

In direct contrast, church treatments are not purchased, and the lack of payment is cited by help-seekers as an indication of authenticity and good intentions. Perhaps even more important, pastors and prophets are keenly aware of the ambivalence many feel about *curandeiros* and stress that the Holy Spirit is an entirely different healing power in continual struggle with the harmful occult forces that traditional healers engage; church healers, they state, are unambiguously on the side of the good and the moral. Since church healers ply the same spiritual terrain as local *curandeiros,* often exorcizing malevolent spirits using local terms and idioms, it is critical that they draw this distinction and harden this boundary. The contrast between the sale of *curandeiro* services and the churches' offer of free healing provides just the opportunity to tap into deepening local anxieties about the morality of accumulation, growing social competition, and the importance of access to cash for survival in the commodifying economy. The changing social environment has provided an opening for church healers to fortify the boundary between their practices and traditional healing. Rapidly widening disparities, and alleged curandeiro complicity in contributing to new inequalities, have brought this contrast into even sharper relief and pastors and prophets have effectively undermined curandeiro legitimacy in the eyes of many.

Perception of efficacy, of course, is a critical determinant of treatment choices, and many of those interviewed sought help from prophet healers after hospital and *curandeiro* treatments were believed to have failed. Most respondents recounted long frustrating periods of seeking help from various sources that included biomedical providers, home remedies, black-market pharmaceuticals, and *curandeiros* before finally turning to church prophets, usually in desperation, to resolve a persistent affliction. Seemingly disparate episodes of illness and other misfortunes among different family members, especially children, are often woven together to reveal the intervention of a "bad spirit," or *espirito mau* in Portuguese.

The Modernity of Traditional Healing

While traditional healing has been celebrated in the international public health world, community attitudes toward *curandeiros* are ambivalent since many healing practices include morally troubling engagements with the spirit world to achieve socially damaging ends such as the enrichment of paying clients at the expense or misfortune of others. *Curandeiros* can potentially harness both the positive and destructive powers of the spirit world—that is, the volatile world of the dead—to cure, bring good luck, send misfortune, or even kill.[2] That witchcraft and occult practices, including healing and sorcery, help individuals manage social position amid new inequalities associated with "modernity" has attracted a renewed interest in witchcraft among Africanists (Kohnert 1996; Maxwell 1995, 1999; Geschiere 1997, 1999; Meyer 1993; Comaroff and Comaroff 1993, 1999; Auslander 1993; Yamba 1997; Englund 1996; Moore and Sanders 2001). As Geschiere (1999, 213) has emphasized, witchcraft can be a leveling force, undermining inequalities in wealth and power, but it can also help individuals accumulate wealth and achieve upward social mobility. He writes, "Witchcraft is both jealousy and success. It is used to kill but also to heal" (Geschiere 1999, 213). Classic anthropology on witchcraft and sorcery emphasized the integration of occult practices with local dynamics of envy, notions of the limited good, misfortune, or good fortune (see discussions in Gluckman 1956; Marwick 1965; Evans-Pritchard 1937; Middleton and Winter 1963).[3] Whether in its power of explanation or in its instrumentality, witchcraft has provided a lens through which to interpret inequalities that both disrupt and animate social life. And as Jean and John Comaroff emphasize, "[W]itchcraft is not simply an imaginative 'idiom.' It is chillingly concrete, its micropolitics all-too-real. As Evans-Pritchard (1937) long ago maintained, its occurrence is explicable only with reference to its particular pragmatics; to the ways in which, in specific contexts, it permits the allocation of responsibility for, and demands action upon, palpable human inequities and misfortunes" (1993, xxvii). Much of the new literature argues that witchcraft and occult practices appear to be increasing in contemporary Africa, at least in part because of their usefulness in responding to new inequalities that emerge with modernity. However, as Moore and Sanders suggest, "[C]ontemporary scholars of witchcraft cast occult beliefs and practices as not only contiguous with *but constitutive of modernity*" (2001, 12, emphasis added).

Curandeiros in Chimoio are vital agents for many in managing individual misfortune, offering social protection, and providing a competitive edge. They have become the focus, not surprisingly, of social anxiety and desire as economic disparities have widened within local communities. The market for these kinds of services has apparently grown as social and economic insecurity has become heightened and the healers themselves, who are usually very poor, have found rewarding ways to ply their trade. Hence the purported increase in, or increased anxieties about, competitive and dangerous forms of sorcery purchased from *curandeiros* in communities such as Chimoio. The implication of *curandeiros* in these morally questionable practices and public unease about their profiteering from the expensive sale of these services has generated a community discourse of distrust that extends well beyond the churches. Poor women are at a special disadvantage in these circumstances, since most are unable to generate any significant cash to pay for protective treatment. Yet they remain in desperate need of spiritual defense given the dangers associated with reproduction in the context of extraordinarily difficult material conditions and dwindling familial support. The evidence presented here suggests that lay members' decisions to join these movements were not experienced or described as a break with tradition. Traditional healing practices had already been transformed to address the afflictions of various confrontations with "modernity" produced by colonialism, the post-independence experiment with socialism, and the civil war. These forces have generated vast changes in social life and healing practices over the past century in the region. In this postwar/post-socialist moment, *curandeiro* practices have adjusted to accommodate local fears and desires incited by "free markets" and state withdrawal from social life. In this sense, the flight to churches in Chimoio appears to be as much a flight from the modernity of traditional healing as it is a break with the past.

Research Methods

Conducted in 2002 and 2003, the interviews described here were collected as part of a larger study of AIC and Pentecostal expansion in the central Mozambican city of Chimoio and its relationship to structural adjustment and deepening social inequality in the region. The research focused on churches in three contiguous periurban *bairros* (neighborhoods) selected for their large populations of residents who represent a broad socioeconomic range and are demographically similar to the rest of the city. The population of the three *bairros* totals over 21,000 people (INE 1998). Ten churches were visited in the *bairros* and recent converts were recruited for more in-depth open-ended illness narrative interviews that centered on health-seeking decisions and experiences that led the respondents to seek treatment from churches. Over eighty interviews were conducted in 2002 and 2003, while dozens of other interviews conducted earlier in 1998 and 2000 in the same *bairros* were reanalyzed in relationship to the central questions in the current research. Pastors, prophet healers, *curandeiros,* health care workers, and other community leaders were also interviewed and church services, healing ceremonies, and baptisms were attended and traditional healing sessions were observed. Thirty randomly selected *bairro* residents who were not members of churches were interviewed to compare experiences and perceptions of healing alternatives. In addition to the collection of illness narratives, a survey of 616 men and women using systematic random sampling was conducted to identify the range of churches in the community, estimate the level of participation in each faith, gather demographic information, and measure social attitudes using a set of questions concerning perceptions of changes in social inequality, social well-being, occult practices, and access to basic services.

Chimoio: Adjustment, Affliction, and the Holy Spirit

Affliction is common and unrelenting among the city's poor. Standard health indicators reveal the impact of severe material deprivation on the majority of the population and the reproductive dangers that poor women face. From 40 percent to 50 percent of children under five are chronically malnourished, cumulative under-five mortality is estimated at nearly 20 percent, and maternal mortality may be as high as 1,000–1,500 per 100,000 (Ulmera et al. 1994; Ministry of Health 1997; UNDP 1998). The city's population has more than tripled since independence in 1975, expanding from about 50,000 to over 170,000 as thousands moved to the city in search of safety during the protracted war with South Africa–backed rebels (known by their Portuguese acronym RENAMO) that finally ended in 1992. Most Chimoio residents and families are peasant-proletarians who combine cash-earning opportunities with subsistence production on small parcels of land called *machambas* outside the city where maize and sorghum are cultivated as staples. Chimoio is a multilingual city: the majority of the population speak Chiteve, Chindau, Chimanica, and other Shona variants. Chisena, Chinhungwe, Shangana, and Tonga are also represented in the population. Portuguese is also widely used by most residents.

In seeking treatment for physical ailments, residents select from a dense array of options across the city. The National Health Service provides biomedical care through the provincial hospital and at several health centers. A private health care clinic opened in the city in the mid-1990s that serves the small emerging elite that can afford the high fees. While most state services are free or charge low fees, many providers reportedly ask for under-the-table payments, a problem that worsened when salaries of health care workers dropped with economic adjustment (Cliff 1991). Pharmaceuticals stolen from clinics and hospitals, including chloroquin and antibiotics, are widely available in outdoor markets or at the homes of nurses and doctors. Hundreds of *curandeiros,* both herbalists and spiritualists, are distributed throughout the city and continue to be widely consulted. The churches have expanded in this medically plural environment; some offer spiritual healing that incorporates local notions of illness causation and others practice prayer healing and laying on of hands.

The Zion churches have become the largest religious category in urban areas in Manica Province, according to the 1997 census, claiming about 30 percent of the population. Nearly 5 percent identified themselves as Protestant/Evangelical, a category consisting mostly of Pentecostals (INE 1999). Since census data were collected in the mid-1990s, it is likely that church participation has expanded even more since then. In contrast, the percentage of urban residents who belong to the Catholic Church has declined from about 30 percent in the 1980 census to 20 percent in 1997.

In the survey of three *bairros* reported here, nearly 45 percent of respondents belonged to churches described as Zionist, Apostolic, or Pentecostal. About 12 percent identified as Zionist, 13 percent belonged to Apostolic churches that use prophetic healing (and are often called Zionists by outsiders), and 20 percent were members of a wide range of Pentecostal churches. Catholics accounted for about 23 percent of the total sample. Gender differences in participation were evident. Nearly 16 percent of all women respondents were members of Zion churches, in contrast to 8 percent of men. Twenty-two percent of women versus

17 percent of men belonged to Pentecostals, while nearly 26 percent of men were members of the Catholic Church, in contrast to only 20 percent of women.

The expansion of AIC and Pentecostal churches in the 1990s gained momentum in part because the Mozambican government loosened its regulation of religious expression, allowing church movements from the southern African region to enter Mozambique and proselytize more freely (Vines and Wilson 1995). Since then, all churches have been able to recruit and mobilize members without the government interference and oversight that characterized the post-independence period in the 1970s and 1980s. However, other faiths dwindled in the 1990s; the rapid growth in AIC and Pentecostal churches is not fully explained by the religious opening of the late 1980s.

As the church movements grew, other sweeping changes in social and economic life were under way in Mozambique. In 1987, a World Bank/IMF structural adjustment program was initiated, even as the war dragged on, that led to privatization of and cutbacks in social services, shredding of social safety nets, arrival of foreign aid, and growing corruption that has spawned rapid class formation and glaring economic disparities over a very short period (Marshall 1990; Cliff 1991; Fauvet 2000; Hanlon 1996). These social and economic changes accelerated further after the fighting ended in 1992. While Mozambique has been hailed for its relatively robust economic growth in the 1990s, benefits have trickled up to a small business elite which has benefited while many Mozambicans remain in absolute poverty (Ministry of Planning and Finance 1998; Hanlon 1996; INE 1998). Accumulation by some is evident around the city, where hundreds of larger cement houses are under construction, satellite dishes and antennae have appeared on many homes, and expensive sport utility vehicles and private luxury cars cruise the streets. In the eyes of many, the new conspicuous consumption and wealth in the city appears to have no visible source or explanation; new wealth is often assumed to be obtained through crime, corruption, practice of sorcery capabilities purchased from corrupt *curandeiros*. Data collected in the survey for this research revealed that nearly 45 percent of respondents felt that their own households had gotten poorer since the war's end, while only 30 percent felt that they had gotten wealthier.

The integration of Mozambicans in this region of the country into market relationships and commoditized economies is certainly not new. Large-scale migration of male laborers to Southern Rhodesia, South Africa, and local plantations over the last century transformed local economies. Bride wealth, known locally as *lobolo,* has long been paid in cash in the area, and cash remuneration to *curandeiros* has reportedly been fairly common for some time, especially in towns and cities. The socialist period after independence brought an alternative version of "modernity" that certainly curtailed market activities, but money was still exchanged for a variety of services, goods, and social transactions. During this period, the war caused immeasurable trauma to all strata of Mozambican society while straining family relationships of reciprocity and mutual aid. While the recent period of free market promotion and privatization constitutes a continuation of social upheaval, it also marks a new and especially intense deepening of the commoditization of social life and social differentiation. A Ministry of Planning and Finance study of poverty and well-being during this period states, "In general the emerging pattern is one of practices gradually evolving away from practices solely based on friendships and communal co-existence and the exchange of labor for labor to those involving monetary transactions" (1998, 312). One must now pay for access to land in spite of new land tenure laws, and even poor smallholders now pay for help in clearing new *machambas*. Subsidies for food prices have been eliminated, and fees (both legal and illegal) for health care and education have been introduced, making cash income increasingly crucial to survival for the vulnerable and social mobility for the ambitious. The cash price of *lobolo* has inflated to the point that many men can no longer pay; they live with their partners without formal marriage status. The commodification of so many aspects of social life has occurred simultaneously with, and helped cause, rapid class formation and conspicuous accumulation of a fortunate few. What distinguishes the current period from both the socialist and colonial epochs is not simply this commoditization and the arrival of modernity (both had already happened in various forms in Chimoio) but rather the rapid *increase* in new local inequalities based primarily on differential access to cash and marked by intensified social and economic insecurity. The desperate need for money has superseded and in some ways dissolved previous social obligations and other sources of reciprocity. It has also raised suspicions about individual accumulation and misfortune beyond the conventional notions of urban "anomie" and social fragmentation.

Increasing social inequality has undermined poor women's economic security in particular, contributing to an expanded sex trade that ranges from full-time sex work around neighborhood bars to casual provision of sexual favors in exchange for cash or goods such as shoes or clothing. The resulting pressure on intrahousehold relationships has produced greater distrust, allegations of adultery, and fear of the spread of sexually transmitted infections, including AIDS. The ensuing moral panic over perceived promiscuity and prostitution has reportedly destabilized relationships, families, and households. One informant stated that many women are joining churches to escape accusations of prostitution made by husbands, family, and neighbors.

The high price of *curandeiro* services has an especially important impact on women in this environment, most of whom have little or no cash income of their own. In the survey, nearly 60 percent of women stated that they had earned no cash income at all in the previous month, in contrast to only 10 percent of men who earned none. Previous research in a nearby community (Pfeiffer, Gloyd, and Li 2001) also demonstrated that men and women normally control separate income streams within households, so that when women lack their own income they can use cash only at the behest of their husbands. Poor women normally must ask their spouses for money to pay *curandeiro* fees, and women are usually accompanied by their husbands for diagnostic consultations for common problems such as infertility or the persistent illness of a child, according to the healers interviewed for this research. The afflictions are often believed to be related to intrahousehold relationships, and several informants stated that when husbands and wives consult *curandeiros* together, the diagnosis nearly always points to spiritual problems in the wives' families or suggests wives' infidelity, perhaps to avoid angering the husband who pays the fees. In contrast, most women interviewees reported seeking help on their own from churches where payment is not demanded; in some cases, their husbands converted later.

Drogas: Sorcery and Inequality in an Age of Adjustment

Traditional healing, specifically "therapy" that engages the spirit/occult world, involves attempts to influence spiritual forces believed to underlie fortune and misfortune, including illness. In this complex moral universe, both extraordinary fortune and misfortune can be viewed suspiciously. Sorcery, vengeful spirits, angry ancestral spirits, and "immoral" behavior such as infidelity are often implicated in experiences of misfortune, including health problems, but spirits can also be manipulated and mobilized for personal gain (Chavunduka 1978; Gelfand 1962; Gelfand, Mavi, Drummond, and Nderma 1985; Bourdillon 1991). When illness is accompanied by unusual symptoms or circumstances or when biomedical interventions fail, a spiritual cause might be considered and a *curandeiro* consulted to exorcise the offending spirits and provide continued protection. Someone who is especially successful and accumulates material wealth and power may also be suspected of engaging the occult world, with the help of a *curandeiro,* for self-promotion and perhaps to harm social competitors.

In Chimoio, dangerous occult practices that are often lumped together with the English term "witchcraft" are roughly divided into two categories of practitioners and activities that resonate quite differently in the new social environment. Witches (*wakoroya* or *varoya* in Chiteve; *feiticeiro/as* in Portuguese) are often women born with an inherited malevolent spirit that can be manipulated to cause terrible misfortune to others through practice of *uroyi,* or the activity of witches (*feitiço* in Portuguese). *Kukamba* and *kuromba* are Chiteve terms for the purchase of sorcery powers from *curandeiros* that can harm one's enemies or provide good fortune and are activated through substances called *mutombo* in Chiteve (translated as *medicamentos* [medicines] or *drogas* [drugs] in Portuguese). But the term "*medicamentos*," or "*mutombo*" is also used in practices that harm others, that send sickness or misfortune. The Portuguese term *feitiço,* or sometimes *fetichismo,* is also heard in reference to this kind of sorcery activity, but a second Portuguese term, *drogar* (literally to use drugs), is more common to distinguish it from "*uroyi.*" The distinction between *feitiçeiro/as* and *drogados* (one who uses drugs) emerged clearly in several questions on social attitudes in the survey for this research. Over 64 percent responded that the use of *drogas* had increased over the last decade, and over 42 percent agreed that it had increased a great deal. In contrast, only 36 percent believed the problem of witches had increased, while nearly 42 percent believed the problem had diminished. The perceived increase in use of *drogas* is broadly shared among church and nonchurch respondents. Occult practices that can be bought and sold in the new economy and that help clients succeed are those people believe have increased in the new economic and social environment.

The exchange of money and the high prices of *curandeiro* services are also linked to an aura of danger surrounding many consultations. Tales abound of corrupt healers who charge outrageous fees, engage in sorcery to harm others or promote good fortune, and enrich themselves by fomenting conflict within families and among neighbors. Treatments often involve an inversion of the moral world in which help-seekers are required to engage in reprehensible activities such as sleeping with one's mother or daughter, engaging in necrophilia, or taking a life to secure occult powers of protection and enrichment. Acts of moral abomination are the source of occult power and require tremendous courage on the part of the help-seeker. The greater the risk taken, the higher the fee and the greater the potential payoff. The demons that are mobilized in these treatment processes are unpredictable, unstable, and extremely dangerous. Paying a *curandeiro* to engage this world to provide protection, gain good fortune, or harm one's social enemies can go wildly wrong and result in descent into madness for the help-seeker or bring misfortune to one's family.

As described elsewhere for Chimoio (Pfeiffer 2002), *curandeiros* function within a complex spirit world where ancestral guardian spirits, *w(v)adzimu* in Chiteve (or *midzimu* in other Shona dialects), can provide protection from spiritual threats if honored properly, usually through ritual beer-brewing and festivities (Chavunduka 1978; Lan 1985; Gelfand 1962; Bourdillon 1991). Severe illness caused by malevolent spirits and sorcery can result from ancestors' withdrawal of protection for failure to follow ritual patterns of respect, "immoral" behavior such as infidelity, and intrafamily conflict. In Chimoio, avenging spirits of murder victims are among the most dangerous since they seek revenge by creating illness, misfortune, or death in the murderer's family (see Bourdillon 1991 and Lan 1985 for descriptions of similar spirits called *ngozi* in Zimbabwe). Intrafamily conflict and tension is also often attributed to the presence of such avenging spirits, called *mpfukwa* in Chimoio. Such spirits can be aroused with the help of a *curandeiro* by a family seeking to avenge the murder of a relative or enforce the return of stolen property or payment of debt. In contemporary Chimoio, a specific category of avenging spirit called *chikwambo* emerged repeatedly in illness narratives of women church recruits, and one pastor referred to a *chikwambo* "epidemic" in Chimoio (Pfeiffer 2002). They are widely believed to be the most dangerous of spiritual afflictions. One set of *chikwambo* spirits was repeatedly mentioned by healers, prophets, and church members—those of migrant workers who had returned to Manica from Zimbabwe or South Africa with money and goods and had been robbed and killed upon arrival.[4] These malevolent shades are the spirits of innocent people who have been maliciously robbed and murdered who then seek revenge on members of the killer's family, sometimes generations later, causing accidents, illness, loss of work, financial calamity, and general misfortune. In order to appease such an avenging spirit, the affected family must pay the spirit back, offering a young daughter to become a "spirit wife," known as *mukadzi we mpfukwa* in Chiteve or *mulheres de espirito* in Portuguese. If behavior by the wife angers the spirit, he can cause infertility, illness, and death. *Mpfukwa* spirits including *chikwambo* can reportedly be manipulated by skilled *curandeiros* for a fee and sent to cause harm to one's enemies.

The State Intervenes

In the 1980s, the Mozambique Association of Traditional Healers, known by the Portuguese acronym AMETRAMO, was established by the government to officially recognize the important role of *curandeiros* in Mozambican society, to collect taxes and fees, and to set price guidelines for services. A typed two-page table on AMETRAMO letterhead enumerates dozens of treatments with their "official" cost using local spirit categories and terms for treatments that help one obtain employment, avoid accidents, contact ancestor spirits, and a range of other common life worries and desires. The list, which was reportedly established to control prices, suggests just how expensive consultations and exorcisms have become. For example, exorcism of a *mpfukwa* spirit costs 350,000 meticais (not including the initial diagnosis consultation), the equivalent of nearly one-half the minimum monthly wage. Many *curandeiros* in the city, however, are distrustful of AMETRAMO and believe it exists merely to tax healers, and the healers interviewed for this research expressed disdain for the organization. Many informants, both church members and nonchurch residents, blamed AMETRAMO for the inflation of *curandeiro* fees, although some suggested that without the table fees would go even higher. A number of informants argued that genuine *curandeiros* are not AMETRAMO members and can be found only in rural areas. The existence of the price list is seen by some as an indication of the organization's spuriousness, suggesting that some in the *bairros* viewed the fee-for-service arrangement implied by the price list with skepticism. It is also difficult to ascertain whether most *curandeiros* actually adhere to the prices on the list. In one healing session observed by the author, a *curandeira* asked for payment for removing an *mfukwa* spirit, then showed the client and the author her copy of the AMETRAMO price list to justify the 350,000-meticais fee she demanded. The thirty interviews with residents not in churches tended to confirm that high fees were often paid to healers and that the perception that fees are inflated is widespread and not merely an accusation made by churches. However, payments to *curandeiros* can sometimes be spread out over time or paid in other items if necessary, such as clothing, chickens, or goats. It is nearly impossible to assess how the higher prices have affected the number of people who consult *curandeiros*. But when interviewed for this research, the Chimoio president of AMETRAMO lamented the huge loss of business among his membership that he attributed to the new churches. Most of the *curandeiros* interviewed for the research also reported a drop in clients.

Money, Efficacy, and Patterns of Resort

In interviews with recent church converts, prophets, pastors, and non-church respondents, the theme of payment and its influence on perception of treatment legitimacy emerged repeatedly. But help-seekers also complained that *curandeiros* incite conflict within families and between neighbors and then demand huge payments to take out offending spirits and provide ongoing protection from spirit threats derived from these conflicts. Most conversion stories recounted extensive periods of help-seeking, often for health complaints of both parents and children. Church membership is often the latest stop in a long sequence of help-seeking for persistent afflictions such as illness, job loss, money loss, health problems of children, and marital difficulties that are often perceived to be linked and caused by a single malign spirit, frequently a *chikwambo* in Chimoio.

Isabel's story is typical and is worth quoting at some length here. She had joined a locally founded church called Nyasha DzaMwari in Chiteve, or Igreja Apostólica Graça a Deus de Moçambique in Portuguese (The Apostolic Church Thanks to God of Mozambique) about three years before the interview. She had been raised as a Catholic in Chimoio, but a series of misfortunes and health problems provoked a sequence of help-seeking choices that ended with fasting and exorcism in the church.

> When I entered this church I had a problem with a bad spirit that was killing my daughter. I went to the hospital when my daughter got sick. My daughter didn't get better because that spirit took away the power of the medicine [*levava aquele medicamento*] in the hospital. I had to come to this church. So here when I arrived, he [the pastor] said this child has a bad spirit and you have to take it out. You have to go to the mountain for three days without eating anything nor drinking water to see if your daughter survives or not. . . .
>
> [My health problems] began a long time ago when I was a child, I always had this problem. . . . I didn't marry, I got really skinny, every day I dreamt of bad things, I didn't want to go to school because of that spirit. At times I didn't even want to take a bath, I only wanted to fight with people, get insulted with people when they did nothing because that spirit gave bad luck [*azares*] in whatever way. . . . I did manage to get married, but my husband that married me, he worked out but my spirit always abused my husband. He began to drink and he lost his job [he was a schoolteacher]. The spirit also attacked my husband. I went to the *curandeiro* but it wasn't possible. . . . The *curandeiro* spoke of the same things [as the church]. "You have a bad spirit" but he didn't manage to take it out, he just took my money. The *curandeiro* said that this bad spirit comes from your grandparents that provoked, killed someone a long time ago. That spirit comes at night to sleep with me. My father also knew about this spirit, but they didn't go to church so they didn't know how to take it out. I didn't know I had the spirit because I was a child, other things hid it from me, but my parents knew. . . . They tried to treat it but it wasn't possible. I conceived a child who was always sick and I went many times [to the *curandeiro*], but now when I began to pray in these churches I saw that going to

curandeiros isn't good because I always went to *curandeiros* and some would say pay a million meticais others 500,000 meticais. I saw that that isn't worth it. I had to come here and pray, since coming here to Nyasha DzaMwari I don't have problems and I don't go to the *curandeiro* anymore.

When you get there [to the *curandeiro*] he has his things; some will shake these things, others sit in their chairs and their spirit starts to come out. He then begins to say "give me some money," maybe 1,000 meticais, you give it to him and he rubs it in his hands. He begins to look at the money, and begins to say, "I'm seeing this and that, I see a spirit that is chasing you but you haven't provoked anyone. Who provoked this spirit are your grandparents. A long time ago this person came from Zimbabwe and had lots of things, so your grandfather killed that person and took those blankets and things. So the spirit of that person who was killed is in your body . . . that spirit is returning to the grandchildren because the grandparents have died, so that spirit is continuing to harass you and you're suffering because of this." To end this problem you have to pay a lot of money to *curandeiros*. You have to bring 500,000 for him to make the spirit go away, but it never works. I had many problems, with children and with me, my husband was drinking a lot and didn't have a job, he just drank. He never contributed to expenses or anything. When he got some money he just drank in the kiosques [small neighborhood bars]. . . . Because I was doing so badly but I always heard and asked about a church called Nyasha dzaMwari. There they have a prophet, when you arrive there if you have a bad spirit they will take it out and you get better, so I began to ask where is this church? . . . When I arrived there the pastor told me these things, he said to end all this you have to pray and this spirit will flee. . . . While it wasn't my body it was because of that spirit that went with me, sucked my blood and I began to pray. I have three years [in the church] and up to now I haven't had any problem. My husband goes to work, he brings home food, I am also working without problems.

Others who described their help-seeking and conversion experiences provided similar accounts. The difficulty of paying for both biomedical and traditional healing was a recurring theme in explaining the choice of church healers. However, in the narratives, the *meaning* of monetary payment to the legitimacy and value of spiritual treatments emerged as a key concern in decision making, as the following selections help illustrate:

I entered this church, Graça Bíblica de Moçambique on January 23, 2000. I went to the church to pray, I saw that to stay at home without praying wasn't helping and when you pray you find a lot of family, your family with the church family, you can get sick, and everyone comes to visit you, so you get a lot of family in the church. . . . I can see now that the church is helping more than when I spent money going to the *curandeiro* to do I don't know what. I was spending a lot of money at the *curandeiro*. . . . 1000 times I'd rather be in the church than spend money for the *curandeiro*. At times you give money to the *curandeiro* when he doesn't do anything, and if you ask for everything in the name of God, God helps. (Woman, Graça Bíblica)

When you go to a *curandeiro* its 600,000, 700,000 meticais . . . just to lie, even for just 50,000 meticais. Because of this people are fleeing. A mother that doesn't work, doesn't do anything [for money] makes a consultation with a healer and pays 50,000, just for a fever. Because of this people are fleeing [*curandeiros*]. (Woman, Apostolic Faith Mission)

Curandeiros always lie that you were born sick, afterward you go there, he says I'll cure you, but you return home, you continue to be sick, a child dies, another child gets sick and dies, so you have to go to the *curandeiro* spending money without any result. (Man, Zion Christian Church)

Church doctrine is relentlessly critical of traditional healers; this could explain the salience of high *curandeiro* fees in explanations so many people in the narratives gave about why they sought help from churches, especially those of women. However, interviews with a wide range of *bairro* respondents who are not church members, including thirty residents and a number of healers themselves, helped confirm that *curandeiro* fees in the city have indeed inflated a great deal. Many nonchurch respondents told of paying millions of meticais over time to handle spiritual afflictions, and healers who were interviewed corroborated the high prices they charged for key treatments. Several interviewees who had not joined churches indicated that they failed to follow through with *curandeiro* treatments after initial consultations because they lacked money. A number of nonchurch respondents stated that in their recent experiences with *curandeiro* treatments they had to cobble together the funds over time from other family members to make the payments.

Bound together with these concerns over payment is a widely shared distrust of *curandeiros* because of the conflict they can incite with their diagnoses and recommended remedies. In interview after interview respondents commented on the dangers that *curandeiros* pose to social and family life. The following selections from interviews are representative.

Curandeiros are not good because they ruin the family, ruin the home, ruin everything. . . . They destroy; when you arrive there and they tell you that the person doing sorcery against you is so and so, if it happens to be your brother, then you believe this and you have to get your nerve up, as soon as you see that brother you get into a conflict [*fica com barrulho*], because of this *curandeiros* are not good. (Man, Zion Christian Church)

I can go to the *curandeiro* and he'll say, Senhor Rungo you're sick and the person doing this to you is your wife, and then love ends. I can give other examples. I arrive there, he says you're sick because your mother did this to you and I start having a conflict with my mother. To avoid this we have to believe in Christ. With the *curandeiro*, you lose money, lose your family, and you lose support. (Man, Apostolic Church of Mozambique)

The problem is with *curandeiros*. Because we don't prohibit medicines. I go to the hospital and they have medicines there and pills and I don't know what else. If he says look, you have a wound here take this medicine and you will get better. We can go to the *curandeiro* but he doesn't talk like that, he begins to say "come here and tell me about your life. So and so hates your family, hates you and gave you this wound. You have to separate from this family or leave that house. . . .

With problems with your neighbor, it comes from that house and you have to resolve the problem with your neighbor family, or whatever family, your wife's family. Your family doesn't like your wife, because of this you're sick. . . ." [B]ecause of this our policy is we don't go to the *curandeiro*. (Pastor, Zion Christian Church)

"We're poor, we come to God without paying": Money and Healing in the Churches

Church prophets and pastors are adept at taking advantage of these concerns over price and payment to contrast themselves with *curandeiros,* whose high fees and socially harmful prescriptions are confirmations of their greed and malicious intent when they sell access to occult powers. Pastors highlighted theological explanations of the importance of free treatment. One pastor (from Nyasha dzaMwari) declared,

> He [Jesus Christ] cured people, took out the bad spirits, he took them out for free, people were saved in the same way we do it here. A person comes with difficult situations and is cured and doesn't provide any reimbursement for that help he received. And because it's free we say the person is saved thanks to God and to thank him we must pray, convert and thank God, adore your God, because he has done this for you and you came to be saved, so you have to recognize God. Its because of this that many people come here, because it's done for free, for this help everyone returns because of this help they received.

A pastor from a Zionist church provided a similar explanation,

> We allow people to go to the hospital, but not the *curandeiro*. Our Bible says, come to me everyone will be saved and no one is going to pay, only by your faith. Afterwards, if a brother [of the church] goes from here to a *curandeiro,* he's going to have his money taken in vain. We're poor, we come to God without paying.

A number of self-declared prophet healers in Chimoio function outside formal congregations, quite like *curandeiros,* charging money to exorcize malignant spirits by invoking the Holy Spirit without requiring their clients to convert. Prophets who charge fees are often dismissed as *curandeiros* by other church leaders; payment and what it represents was the defining criteria people used to determine whether a prophet healer was genuine. One pastor stated, "There exist some prophets that work for money, whatever money. This is like a *curandeiro* and we have a conflict with *curandeiros.* For example, we receive our brothers [recruits] with a health problem, an illness, we treat them but they don't pay anything. . . . But for us, our religion doesn't allow it, cure a person and after demand payment, because we work for God." Payment indicates that the provider is not working with God's interests in mind; thus, the provider's claims that he or she has access to the healing power of the Holy Spirit must be false. Clients who pay have not genuinely converted, so healing cannot be successful. One Zion Christian Church pastor stated, "A person going down that road is not praying for salvation but is just doing it for their well-being of their life and nothing more." Church pastors speak of a distinction between the world, *o mundo*, where one pays for everything including healing, and life inside the church. But when "one goes to God it's free and you get better. I had to leave 'the world' to go in front of Jesus. . . . When you pay you are no longer saying that you are with Jesus but you're in the 'world.'" Genuine healing in the Holy Spirit requires conversion, faith, and a moral life; payment for such a transformation is anathema to church doctrine.

It can be appropriate for a client to offer a prophet an item, even money, in a spirit of thankfulness and generosity. One prophet healer stated, "The *curandeiro* demands payment, because where he went to get his powers he had to pay, but when you go to a prophet you don't pay anything. You go to the mountain [to fast]; you don't pay. Now spiritual power is not purchased with money, you treat a person, he gets cured, later he might feel that he wants to give me something like a shirt or some corn flour, that's his choice, but you can't ask him to pay." Transforming the transaction into a sale appears to undermine the moral legitimacy of the healer, the client's intentions, and the healing activity itself. The difference between the sale and the gift parallels the distinction between the "world" and life in the church. And it is this difference that pastors and prophets highlight to mark a boundary as clearly as possible between the morally ambiguous *curandeiro* and the morally pure world of the church.

Money gathered through tithing and collections within the congregations plays an important and dynamic role in the social life of the churches, but it functions very differently from payments made to *curandeiros* or prophet healers. Members are often asked to contribute 10 percent of their earnings (*dízimos* in Portuguese) to their church, and some individual members may contribute a great deal of money over time. In Sunday service collections, a basket is normally passed and members are asked to donate 1,000 meticais if they have it, though many do not. These funds are then passed forward to the church leadership and usually end up with the pastor or deacons to be spent on church materials. But these contributions are believed by lay members to support the collective and are experienced as a form of redistribution; they are never linked directly to healing practices. One Zion Christian Church pastor explained, "A gift is a gift that you take out for your God. That money isn't to be given to somebody [*alguém*]; it's only to be used in the church, the group, if it's necessary to buy a bench, or whatever the church needs." In the women's groups, modest financial support is often provided to those in need. One woman member said, "We normally help when someone is suffering, they [women in the church] come to help with whatever they can in money. The church will take out an amount from the [church] mothers, they take the money and give it to the mother; even if it's 10–20,000 meticais it's a lot. We have a lot of support." In most cases, the final collection during services is handed to the recipient in full view of the congregation and the total is announced. However, while this mutual financial assistance appears to provide a kind of safety net, the circulation of money in many congregations also constitutes an ever-present, lurking danger that threatens to destabilize the collective. Not surprisingly, the defining characteristic of a false prophet or pastor is his theft of church funds or profiting from treatment of health problems. Most pastors handle all transactions with extreme care to avoid appearances of impropriety.

Many non-Pentecostals in the community are skeptical of the recent proliferation in the number of churches and believe that entrepreneurial pastors recognize the potential to make money and found new churches to make a living or gain sexual access to women. Some of those interviewed believed that pastors drew believers in, especially women, through free treatment but then extracted funds slowly over time through tithes and contributions. A majority of the twenty-five pastors interviewed for this project were unemployed. The tendency of the churches to split off to form new congregations often stems from accusations of disillusioned members around theft of church funds.

Discussion

The influence of rising *curandeiro* fees on treatment choices and conversion to churches clearly extends beyond the basic price barriers the fees create for the poor; motives for resort to church healers cannot be simply reduced to economic considerations. In fact, many church members may contribute more to their church over time than they might otherwise spend on *curandeiro* fees. If high *curandeiro* fees were a barrier, one might expect prices to eventually come down in response to declining demand, and indeed they may have in some instances. However, the church movements in Chimoio have so effectively demonized the *curandeiros* that the growing aversion is not simply a response to high cost but a reaction to what the rising prices imply about the services rendered. Under these conditions even declining fees may not effectively shift client preferences away from churches back to *curandeiros* for the treatment of illness and misfortune. Rather, the rising fees in the new environment raise troubling questions about the morality of accumulation by healers and their clients in the context of widening local economic disparities and the misfortunes of so many. This creates social dilemmas for clients seeking new prosperity and combating persistent misfortunes, whether in the form of illness, infertility, job loss, financial struggles, or familial conflict. The conspicuous sale of *curandeiro* services for high profit appears to be one of the most troubling aspects of traditional healing for many help-seekers in this environment; access to malevolent and powerful occult forces is being sold to enrich the provider, often at great expense and danger to others.

A number of informants asserted that in earlier historical periods, payment to *curandeiros* represented a modest gesture of thanks rather than a purchase. The dramatic inflation of fees in the postwar period suggests that some healers are selling their skills for apparently excessive profit, and the most profitable treatments, such as *drogas*, may be the most socially dangerous. The perception that *curandeiros* increasingly help mostly male clients to *drogar*, or engage in sorcery practices for good fortune and to harm others, recasts healers as agents of social conflict that specialize in the management of malignant spiritual forces. *Curandeiros* apparently alienate many poor women more than they heal amid declining economic security, destabilized households, and perceived infidelities. On the other hand, the high fees also confirm that *curandeiros* remain an important source of support for many Mozambicans who have access to the cash, especially men seeking fortune and protection. In this way, "traditional" healers remain, for some, as relevant and necessary to surviving and prospering in "modern" Chimoio as church prophets.

Pastors and prophets have effectively used these concerns over payment and sale of services to mark a clear boundary and contrast themselves with the morally suspect healing practices of many *curandeiros*. This contrast and hardened boundary is serving them well. The Pentecostal message brings a different and dynamic healing experience within a new collectivity that is well suited to the experience of marginalization, spiritual danger, and moral uncertainty. In this sense, the new, local, and all-too-real micropolitics (Comaroff and Comaroff 1993) of stark and growing inequalities, both within and among households, remain the focus of help-seeking processes that are filling the churches.

Recognition of the importance of these dynamics to the growth of AIC and Pentecostal churches does not preclude consideration of a wide range of other influences on these overdetermined movements. A host of crucial and vexing questions remain. As inequality worsens, do the new churches mediate rapid social differentiation or help constitute new class identities and even resistance to new experiences of marginalization? Alternatively, how might they do both? Are the new church collectivities nostalgic reconfigurations of rural communities shattered by colonialism and war or novel forms of adaptation to a new political economy? How do church healing practices themselves both recall and contrast with certain aspects of traditional healing? For example, both often include use of treated water to cleanse help-seekers of malignant avenging spirits; but church healers, unlike *curandeiros*, counsel avoidance of confrontation with social antagonists. In what ways does the quality of the religious conversion experience itself attract new members, above and beyond perceived efficacy in treating common health problems or obtaining new social support? How do the new churches contribute to or mediate new intrahousehold and extrahousehold gender inequalities?

To be sure, there are pastors who speak of breaking with tradition, pastors whose imaginations are captured by the international, even global, reach of Pentecostal ideas. A perceived contrast between the poverty of tradition and the prosperity of modernity seems to resonate with some church leaders in Chimoio. However, interviews with lay members reveal that other, more local concerns and motivations for choosing churches over healers to address their misfortunes and hopes may underlie rapid church growth. Rather than situating the success of Pentecostal churches within the generalized and supposedly inevitable processes of transition from an "invented" tradition to global modernity, it is argued here that the recent turn to the Holy Spirit, in Mozambique at least, underscores the social costs of the current free market experiment; an experiment that was neither inevitable nor synonymous with modernity. The current moment is an especially important one in central Mozambique, not because modernity and globalization have just arrived but because new forms of power relations, class struggles, and market forces have jarred these communities in different ways once again. The rapid withdrawal of safety nets, growing inequality, and new pathways to accumulation that characterize this version of modern peripheral capitalism have confounded and distorted previous healing approaches and provided new opportunities for alternatives.

Notes

This research has been made possible by individual research grants from the National Science Foundation (BCS-0135860) and the Wenner-Gren Foundation for Anthropological Research (Grant 6784). Additional logistic support was provided by Health Alliance International in Mozambique and the Manica Province Health Directorate.

1.   Because their central tenets and practices are similar, this chapter treats AICs and Pentecostal Churches as overlapping segments of a general Pentecostal movement. They are similar in their incorporation of key tenets of Pentecostalism, including belief in the healing power of the Holy Spirit, the authority of New Testament scripture, ritualized speaking in tongues, ceremonies of baptism, and spiritual explanations for misfortune and illness (Cox 1995). Both groupings of churches trace their histories to the same early Pentecostals.
      There are important differences, however. Some of the Pentecostals in Chimoio have international links to global networks, while AICs by definition are linked only to regional groups and are often founded locally. The major perceived distinction between the AICs and more mainstream Pentecostals in Chimoio is the AIC's use of prophet healers to communicate with the spirit world in the healing process in ways that are often called syncretistic. For mainstream Pentecostals, such as the African Assembly of God, this prophet healing recalls African traditional healing and is frowned upon. Instead, pastors use prayer healing (summoning the Holy Spirit) and the laying on of hands to heal. However, some well-known international Pentecostals in Chimoio, such as the Apostolic Faith Mission, have recently begun prophet healing, perhaps as a strategy to gain more members. Two sets of AICs, the Zionists and the Apostolics, use prophetic healing (see extended discussion in Pfeiffer 2002). The influence of Pentecostalist ideas among AICs can be traced historically to the arrival of Pentecostals from the U.S.-based Apostolic Faith Mission and Zionist evangelists from Alexander Dowie's Zion City, Illinois (who increasingly adopted Pentecostal principles) to South Africa in the early twentieth century (see Cox 1995; Comaroff 1985; Sundkler 1961). The terms "Apostolic" and "Zion" appear in the names of many AICs, but it is often difficult to determine historical linkages because of the ten-

dency of churches to split and the local founding of new independent congregations.

2. Evans-Pritchard (1937) famously contended that witchcraft involved an inherited ability and spirit while sorcery could be learned or purchased in many African contexts. This basic distinction appears in Chimoio as well.

3. As Moore and Sanders remind us, Evans-Pritchard's view differed with that of the structural-functionalist Manchester School (Gluckman, Marwick, Turner and others), which reduced witchcraft to a "social strain-gauge" and pressure valve that helped maintain social homeostasis. See further discussion in Moore and Sanders (2001, 6–13).

4. Maxwell (1995) mentions *chikwambo* spirits in Zimbabwe, and some ethnography on Shona healing in Zimbabwe refers to *chikwambo nyangas,* who are consulted by clients seeking retribution from someone who has harmed them or failed to pay back debt (Gelfand et al. 1985).

5 Transnational Images of Pentecostal Healing: Comparative Examples from Malawi and Botswana

Rijk van Dijk

Recent footage of a healing ritual in Mvumbwe, a small village near the city of Blantyre in Malawi, appeared to demonstrate an element of stasis and boundedness that many similar phenomena tend to display. The footage, produced by a student of mine, showed the healing practice of the prophetess Maria ya Mvumbwe, a well-known spiritual healer who I met ten years ago treating patients at the same location and with the same set of symbolic repertoires, medicines, helpers, music, and dancing. Her healing practice consisted then, as it does now, of two different and very distinct moments: the first setting is indoors and focuses on bringing out the avenging spirit and a second setting, outdoors, features medicines of various kinds that are administered once the first period of treatment starts to show positive results. In the first part, the client stands in the center of a circle of dancing and singing assistants who move around the sufferer during the healing ritual. The person in the middle will slowly and gradually go into a trance. His or her body will start to shiver and shake and the movements of the head and arms become wilder as time passes and the circling of the assistants continues. In the meantime, Maria approaches the patient at regular intervals and, tapping her fingers on the person's chest, shouts "*Ndani, ndani, ndani?!*" ("Who is there? What is your name?"). Persistent questioning during the ceremony urges the spirit residing in the person to come out and reveal its identity. Maria expects a name with a biblical connotation such as Peter, Mark, David, or Jacob to be whispered in her ear. The ritual will then unfold with Maria reading aloud passages from the Bible and tapping the person on the head, the chest, and the back with the Bible. The person will then go outside to receive medicines that are meant to tranquilize both the physical body and the spirit that is manifesting itself in the person's life.

The striking element of the indoor setting is not so much its syncretic nature, which in itself is an all-too-well-known example of symbolic border-crossings of a deeply multifaceted nature that commonly characterize rituals of this kind.

Instead, a great deal of attention is paid to the person so that he or she does not move during the singing and clapping, which can last for many hours. The footage of my student showed how the person in the center—with his body shaking violently—appeared to be choking on something while Maria continued to tap his chest. In the end, the man began to dribble and even started to throw up. However, this was to no avail, as the cathartic moment never arrived and the shouts of "*Ndani, ndani*" did not produce the desired name. The man had not moved an inch, a feature of the ritual that even a decade ago struck me as distinctive and which has not changed since.

Obviously, in symbolic terms, what Maria ya Mvumbwe displays here is the dialectic of movement versus petrifaction, of being blocked and of even choking on spirits that have immobilized the person. The person is perceived as being "stuck" (*ku tsaka* or *ku tsama*), and by announcing the name of the (biblical) spirits—names that clearly originate elsewhere and demonstrate a kind of transgressive potential of Christianity—the person is able to overcome the obstructions that are affecting his or her life. The subject of this particular ceremony declared himself "stuck" because his small business of bringing goods into Malawi from neighboring countries was no longer flourishing and something was blocking prosperity and success.

It is interesting that Maria ya Mvumbwe's ritual practices and those of a range of healers and prophetesses like her are emerging amid a plethora of new Christian charismatic movements in Malawi (see van Dijk 1992, 1995, 1998, 1999; Von Doepp 1998; Englund 2001) that emphasize their significance for personal healing and prosperity and their capacity to move about so as to be relevant in the transnational—even global—domain. Most of these are of a Pentecostal orientation. Contrary to the image of stasis, Pentecostal churches proclaim that faith is capable of "moving things" and can "move mountains" and is therefore able to put persons and even the entire nation on the road to prosperity. Pentecostalism perceives itself as being a "movement" in the most literal sense of the word. Pentecostal churches and all the activities they organize in various parts of the country, tellingly termed "crusades," have become very popular over the last two decades. They indeed display an attractive type of energetic liveliness in their meetings through dancing, music, and the movement of bodies as members receive the healing power of the Holy Spirit. In addition, beyond this significance for people in a local setting, these churches stress their importance for the nation as a whole as they address the predicament of the state in moral terms in prayers for the nation. Personal healing, through the laying on of hands and the deliverance of evil forces in one's life, is just one element of the way in which the Pentecostal faith is thought to be relevant to the healing of larger cultural and national wholes. They also move beyond the boundaries of the nation and seek to become relevant for other countries in the region.

This chapter[1] explores the rise of these forms from the perspective of religious mobility (see also Werbner 1989). Although they share some of the same features as the sessions of healers such as Maria ya Mvumbwe in terms of the personal problems they tackle, the songs and rhythms they use, and the use of the Bible as a universal panacea, there are a number of remarkable differences between the two healing modalities that can be traced to different perceptions of cultural boundedness. Maria's healing practices and her use of herbal medicines relate to a wider and more regionally embedded cultural repertoire. Although these regional repertoires of healing exist across national borders and have, perhaps since precolonial times, maintained their significance for many citizens of these present-day nation-states, the question is whether these healing practices are transnational in the full sense of the word.

A growing anthropological literature sees the newly emerging Pentecostal churches as quintessentially transnational, particularly in the way they adopt a global frame of reference for their ideological underpinnings and the way they are able to move from one country to another with a highly uniform set of healing practices. Little information is available in terms of how precisely this transnational aspect is relevant for their healing practices. The question is what these churches actually transcend and how the ways in which they distance themselves from the nation in order to overcome its limitations has relevance to their healing practices. In the anthropological literature, too much is taken for granted regarding the transnational features of these churches, particularly where the concept relates to the creation of transcultural religious styles that may facilitate identity constructs that seem to have global or cosmopolitan dimensions. Most studies of transnational movements take a predominantly geographical perspective in defining the term (see Basch, Schiller, and Blanc-Szanton 1994; Vertovec 2001; Portes 1998, 217–218). As Rudolph and Piscatori (1997) and Beyer (2001) have proposed, the term transnationalism implies a focus on how religious movements can transcend national identities, thus adopting a critical distance from the state of the nation in order to critique its shortcomings and tribulations. While such sociological studies can indicate the transcending quality of transnational religions, little ethnography is available on how transcultural identities are actually formed and what the healing practices they offer signify in day-to-day contexts of social reality.

This chapter highlights the fascination that exists in Botswana society for forms of healing that are perceived to originate from elsewhere and that generate awe and respect precisely because of their capacity to become embedded locally. Moreover, it appears that there is a wide interest in religious forms that come from abroad, such as the healing practices of Maria ya Mvumbwe, which are perceived to originate in Malawi. By exploring the position of a newly established Pentecostal church in Gaborone that originally came from Malawi, the significance of this transnational element to the success of Pentecostal churches can be fruitfully analyzed. This Pentecostal church appears to have opened up a much wider horizon for its practices as it became dominated and heavily influenced by immigrants to Botswana from West Africa, Ghana in particular. In this development, the church demonstrates the capacity of its healing practices to transcend all sorts of geographical and cultural borders and in the process to gain power and public appeal. While the nation-state is becoming the context of the changing fortunes of social mobility, and this is very much the case in present-day Botswana, churches of this kind and their forms of healing appear to be capable of integrating religious forms that have appeal precisely because they are not "stuck" within the nation or the region. Those who are drawn to powerful elements of religious practice want to become part of a wider identity that qualifies being Malawian or being a Motswana, and goes beyond what is already available on a regional basis. The way in which this shaping of extraregional identities is related to the appeal of transnational forms of healing is at the heart of the analysis of this kind of Pentecostalism in present-day Botswana.

Pentecostal Healing and Transnationalism in the Region

The study of the rise of Pentecostalism in Africa in recent years has been informed by a fascination with processes of globalization that has marked the social sciences. Pentecostalism is often placed in the context of living in a global world characterized by "flows"—that is, an unhampered and unfettered movement of people and ideas around the globe (Basch, Schiller, and Blanc-Szanton 1994; Appadurai 1996; Meyer and Geschiere 1999). Pentecostalism is often regarded as a significant form of globalization. This specific form of emotional Christianity has enjoyed an almost inexorable spread worldwide. Produced by influential preachers such as Hagin, Roberts, Swaggart, and Bonnke, authors such as Poewe (1994), Hexham and Poewe (1997), and Gifford (1994, 1998) see it as having landed locally. Regions such as Africa and Latin America presumably receive the flows and waves of new Pentecostal groups from America as if the world was borderless (Corten and Marshall-Fratani 2001; see also Beyer 1994). Global Pentecostal organizations use a wide range of links to Africa to introduce their ideas, and the local fascination with what arrives from a "global" world on the doorstep, for instance through the use of the modern media, apparently does the rest (see Hackett 1998). Hence, the new Pentecostal movements which are springing up in great numbers in Africa are often interpreted as an example of globalization par excellence. Too often, however, their transnational mode of operation is confused with their global aspirations and vice versa. While many of these groups have been inspired in their religious ideology and ritual practice by what has arrived on their doorstep through international evangelical and Pentecostal activity, this homogeneity may not necessarily be central to the position these churches take vis-à-vis nation-states and the particular way in which identities are forged that transcend their borders and their national identity projects.

In the southern African region, almost every country has witnessed the rise of this popular brand of Christianity. In Malawi, new Pentecostal movements began to operate among youth and students in the mid-1970s, usually as small fellowships with a highly charismatic and ecstatic orientation. These churches eventually developed into full-fledged megachurches such as the Living Waters Church, which was founded by the well-known pastor Stanley Ndovi.[2] These churches stress spiritual healing, speaking in tongues, crusades, vigils, and above all a "born-again" type of identity change. Similar movements also began to attract large followings in other countries in the region such as Zambia and Zimbabwe (see Gifford 1998; Maxwell 1998).

The arrival in the region of these charismatic forms of Christianity was seen as the result of global outreach by groups from the United States, the UK, or South Africa that were apparently successful in gaining access to the hearts and minds of many by organizing large-scale "crusades" and "rallies for Jesus." Reinhard Bonnke toured the region in the 1980s, as did others from the West, including famous Pentecostal preachers from within Africa (Gifford 1998). Well-known Nigerian evangelist Emmanuel Eni's 1992 visit to Malawi was widely covered in the press. Pan-African Pentecostalist Mensah Otabil from Ghana visited a number of countries in the region from the end of the 1980s up to 1996. While these movements and churches were initially interpreted as right-wing forces preaching an otherworldliness to the often impoverished masses (i.e., a politically conservative force in society that was often supported by the post-independence regimes, see Gifford 1991), over time it became clear that this view was too one-sided.

First, if Pentecostalism was a new form of "religious imperialism" in which Western right-wing religious groups began to dictate to people in Africa what to believe and how to worship, how could one then explain the South-South spread of Pentecostalism whereby groups from Brazil, such as the Universal Church of the Kingdom of God, have made their presence felt in countries such as Malawi and Botswana? Second, the emerging well-educated middle classes have appeared to be increasingly interested—if not fascinated—by Pentecostal ideology. Their attraction to Pentecostalism is only partly fed by a desire to come close to globally circulating ideas of the modern person or conservative liberal ideals relating to identity, style, and appetites. To a large extent the decision to become a born-again appears to be based on the desire to create a distance from local cultural traditions and obligations, to disentangle from kinship structures and responsibilities, and to create a critical awareness of ritual practices that relate to healing and protection. In other words, the rise of Pentecostalism in a country such as Malawi is as much informed by a critical dialogue of continuity versus discontinuity with regard to local cultural traditions and circumstances as it is structured to embrace a globally circulating discourse that happened to arrive on the doorstep of the emerging middle classes.

Third, and perhaps most important in the field of healing, it is clear that although a global Pentecostal rhetoric and ritual practice is alluded to in these new churches, they often relate their rhetoric and practice to a regionally specific history of Pentecostal healing repertoires. In the southern African region, older Pentecostal predecessors to these new churches existed that often included healing practices that syncretically came from a variety of "traditional" healing idioms. These included the treatment of patients with a range of substances, such as water, oil, herbs and roots, and the like, and could include a kind of clientelistic approach to the leader-healers of these churches. The new Pentecostal leaders and their followers often claim to be "charismatics" by way of distinguishing themselves from the earlier Pentecostal churches. Eager to distance themselves from local traditions of healing, they express rigid ideas about why practices of the *nganga* should be declared demonic and deceitful and how veneration of ancestors should be rejected as something that ensnares the individual in a world of devilish powers.

Nevertheless, these Pentecostal churches do not reject the existence of the powers of spirits, witchcraft, and ancestors as mere superstition. Instead, they declare that these powers are relevant to a person's success and prosperity in life. But at the same time, a discourse of superiority emphasizes the power of the Holy Spirit, speaking in tongues, and prayer healing as a way of overcoming these dangers. The way in which these new churches deal with the kind of forces that are capable of besieging the individual and the problems he or she faces because of their existence—from physical problems to other matters of misfortune such as unemployment, divorce, or bad luck—has changed considerably. Prayers, deliverance, and fasting have been introduced as the main "techniques" to achieve healing and prosperity. Herbs, water, and other substances are unanimously declared sinful and devilish. This has become the most significant marker of differentiation between Pentecostal churches and all kinds of (prophetic) healing churches in the region.

A further element in the growing disparity between the spirit-healing churches and the new Pentecostal churches became the Pentecostals' emphasis on conversion in conjunction with an increasing concern about the clientelistic nature of their church leaders' healing practices. Healing became less and less based on a "come and get it" principle but was increasingly seen as truly effective for the person only after he or she had converted. Some churches maintain so-called deliverance ministries that operate at certain hours to offer spiritual help to anybody who stops by, but the actual purpose of such sessions is to stress the notion that the root cause of evil and misfortune can be addressed only after an interested individual has shown visible signs of a full commitment to the church, its leader, and its creeds. Conversion by becoming "born again" signifies an act of healing that first deals with the past and then extends beyond the personal into wider circles of social interaction. A number of recent publications on Pentecostalism in Africa demonstrate how Pentecostal churches are profoundly interested in inspecting an individual's past as a possible source of generational curses (see van Dijk 1998, 2001a; Meyer 1998). In Malawi, the phrase for being "born again" (in the vernacular *kubadwa mwatsopano*) literally means being born in the now as a way of creating a distance from life before conversion in which all kinds of powers may have existed, for good or for evil, but which now should be discarded.

In the healing practices of the new Pentecostal churches in southern Africa, there is little room for ambiguity regarding ancestral powers as a cause of personal suffering. While born-again persons acknowledge these powers and their effectiveness in causing suffering, they are expected to demonstrate that they are "conquerors" who have gained victory in spiritual battles and has moved to "higher grounds" where these forces can no longer reach (the often-heard expression in Malawian Pentecostalism is: "We are more than conquerors!"). This mastery of one's life should transpire in all sorts of ways, particularly with regard to certain common problems of everyday life. Those who appear to have lost control over their lives, for instance due to alcohol abuse, frequently turn to leaders and deliverance ministers in Malawi and Botswana. Alcohol abuse in these countries has risen to unimaginable proportions, particularly in the urban centers, due to changing patterns of consumption and leisure and images of masculinity that see the ability to buy and drink bottled beer and distillates as a symbol of manhood, independence, and consumer power. Pentecostal churches preach a message of social healing that includes deliverance from the demon of alcohol and emphasizes responsibility for household matters. Similar messages of social healing focus on marital relations (the man as the head of the nuclear family), sexuality and the prevention of extramarital affairs (in Malawi mocked in Pentecostal circles as *kyenda-yenda*, "to walk around" with girls), or the treatment of children, the elderly, and family obligations. They also emphasize the importance of giving one-tenth of one's net income to the church; this stresses responsibility to community.

Healing of relations that transcends the level of the individual is present in Pentecostal ideology regarding specific cultural matters. Pentecostal church leaders encourage members to replace ancestral rituals and cultural practices relating to births, weddings, and funerals with Pentecostal ones in the hope that this will create a critical distance from the local culture. In many churches, members give public "testimonies" that recount how they ran into difficulties with elderly relatives when arranging funerals or weddings and when discussing the serving of alcoholic drinks and the pouring of libations to honor the ancestors. Church leaders strongly discourage visits to local *asing'anga* because their powers relate to the world of medicines and herbs and a nocturnal world of spirits which, from the Pentecostal point of view, may be helpers of Satan bent on leading people into demonic contacts and contracts to pursue wealth, success, and prosperity. Pentecostal healing rituals often stress participation in prayer sessions where congregations seek the ecstatic and protective outpouring of the "blood of Jesus" and leaders practice laying on of hands in the hope that the Holy Spirit will descend onto the person. This spirit is decidedly not of ancestral origin and because it comes directly from God is superior to any of the local deities and spirits that may influence a person's well-being. Pentecostalists place a great deal of faith in the power of calling out the name of Jesus, particularly when someone feels threatened by demonic forces of evil or witchcraft. They believe that calling out the name of Jesus in a loud voice, especially at night when vulnerability to such attacks is at its highest, will cause witches and spirits to become "stuck" or "paralyzed" on the doorstep of a house or bedroom, unable to move until daybreak. It is in this sense that the healing politics of Pentecostalism—that is, the way it positions itself vis-à-vis local cultural traditions—acquires a highly personalized and singular relevance. It is capable of turning every believer into a person who has acquired the power to confront evil forces, powers that all too often originate from the domain of (kinship) sociality.

This is not to say that in countries such as Malawi, where Pentecostalism has developed in the larger urban areas and a relationship has developed between Pentecostalism and an urban lifestyle, its ideological discourse and healing practices remain limited to the level of the individual or the cultural. Leaders have begun to speak out on social issues more forcefully over the last few years and some have become national figures who spread their message in the public domain through the modern media. Leaders have begun addressing the situation of the nation-state, sometimes critiquing governments for their policies, for example, the tendency of governments to recapture cultural heritage for the purpose of nation-building. Often an analytical distinction is made between the nation and the state to present ideas about the Christianization of the nation. For example, many of the churches organize "prayers for the nation" and call for divine protection of the nation against the state and its often-despised policies. In rare cases, Pentecostal leaders have even attempted to mediate in political conflicts and act on behalf of the interests of the state. In Malawi, for instance, charismatic leader Madalitso Mbewe organized a "prayer breakfast" attended by political leaders that included President Bakili Muluzi and the leaders of some of the Muslim communities in the country during the 1999 general election. This Pentecostal leader managed to bring parties together and strike a conciliatory tone in the discussions and prayers at a time when Malawi was becoming increasingly troubled by political and religious tensions. Mbewe became well known for managing to achieve something the mainline Christian churches in the country had been unable to do.

This underscores the point that although the impetus for the formation of most Pentecostal churches comes from outside the country and has global dimensions, the reasons for their rapid proliferation have more to do with local circumstances and local cultural traditions. The combination of the image of the believer as a modern individual capable of creating distance from local culture and Malawian Pentecostalism's revisioning of the nation-state project appeal greatly to an up-and-coming middle class. This group, which is often better educated and aspires to well-paid positions in the rapidly retrenching economy, perceives Pentecostalism as a liberal ideology that critically engages both the authority of the family, including the family elders and the obligations of kinship, and the authority of the state. In Malawi, it is this group that cried foul when the Muluzi government decided that all meat sold in stores and supermarkets should be *halal*. Pentecostal churches also adamantly oppose the policies of mainline Christian churches that pursue "enculturation" by introducing certain elements of African traditions into their liturgy. They promote an image of bravery when Pentecostal leaders and members venture into dangerous domains to proselytize. In the 1970s and 1980s, this meant flaunting government regulations, for instance by moving across the border into RENAMO-held territories in Mozambique with the aim of spreading the gospel. Nowadays many

Pentecostals perceive it as a courageous move when a leader goes into Muslim areas to try to convert the people living there. Transcending the level of the individual to heal the nation often takes on conflicting dimensions, a conflict the leaders in particular feel they have every moral right to engage. Neither at the individual level nor at the level of the nation do Pentecostalists perceive healing as a harmonious process. However, wanting to become "healed" from local cultural traditions and from the effects of state cultural policies does not mean an automatic embrace of the global, as if Pentecostalism offers a kind of cosmopolitanism which would allow members to escape from local conditions and circumstances.

The final level in understanding the significance of the rise of spiritual healing in the hundreds of Pentecostal churches that have emerged in the past two or three decades is the transnational. A number of these churches, unlike the so-called spiritual/prophetic healing types of churches, began adding terms such as "global," "international," or "world" to their names, and many have in fact tried to live up to these promises. This is how two Pentecostal churches from Malawi have ended up in Botswana; study of them clarifies what it means to move beyond what Malkki (1995) termed a "national order of things." These two churches—the Bible Live Church International (BLC) of the Malawian pastor Enoch Sitima and the Ghanaian-led but Malawi-based Christ Citadel International Church (CIC)—settled in Botswana's capital city, Gaborone, in the early 1990s. Both quickly attracted middle-class urbanites and benefited from the increasing popularity of Pentecostalism in Botswana, as evidenced by the growth and public presence of a range of other Pentecostal churches. The churches attracted a highly varied membership of nationals from different countries who had settled in the city as international labor migrants from neighboring countries such as Zambia, Zimbabwe, Swaziland, and Malawi but usually also from farther afield in Africa—particularly from Ghana and Nigeria. Local Batswana, therefore, tend to be only one group within the multinational and multicultural makeup of these churches, and in many cases they form a minority. The churches clearly demonstrate their transnational element; for instance, they display the flags of all their members and deliberately use English instead of Setswana, the local language. Furthermore, the cultural styles and traditions of church rituals, such as births, weddings, or funerals, try to downplay differences and instead offer a format with which all cultural orientations feel comfortable.

This strategy applies to spiritual healing in particular, where church leaders find themselves confronted with many distinct cultural practices and cosmological notions of evil, misfortune, and witchcraft. It is interesting that church leaders and prayer-healers rarely appear to be interested in the specific nature of such problems; they do not investigate the root cause of these issues and usually offer a kind of universal panacea for what, in general terms, they refer to as demonic powers that lurk behind unfortunate circumstances. The most important moments of healing in the day-to-day affairs of these churches are the hours for deliverance, which tend to take two different forms. One form of deliverance runs like an ordinary church service in the sense that people are gathered for prayer, preaching, singing, and worshipping; the other involves more direct, face-to-face contact with the healer and/or leader. In the first form, people approach the altar to receive a laying on of hands by the leader, an event that can be repeated several times during the meeting depending on the size of the group and the attention the healer or leader is able to devote to each person individually. Usually the healer will approach the person presenting him or herself at the pulpit and, while singing and dancing goes on, the person is invited to whisper in the leader's ear and describe the problem he or she is facing. Direct physical contact then follows, during which it is considered essential that the leader forcefully touch the person's head while engaging in ecstatic prayer. The result is what is commonly known in Pentecostal circles as being "slain in the Spirit," which indicates a powerful entrance by the Holy Spirit into the person's *da-sein;* an experience considered to be destabilizing to such an extent that the person stumbles and falls backward. This signals that the person has become "loosened" and is now free of the tightening and petrifying grip demons had over his or her life. To make sure that no one is injured in the process, helpers stand behind the person to catch them as they fall. The person is gently laid on the ground, where he or she will stay, usually for a couple of minutes, to recover from the apparent shock therapy, an experience that is sometimes so emotional that it makes people weep. Women are covered up to ensure that decency is maintained throughout the process. Those persons who appear to be moved by the experience to such an extent that they remain in a kind of possessed state after they have been laid on the ground are taken outside, as states of frenzy always produce an uneasy ambiguity about what is actually causing such uncontrolled behavior.

The individualized form of deliverance is far more private and intense. While the process of touching the head remains the same and the entering of benevolent powers into the person's existence is similar, a major difference is the amount the leader or the healer knows about the problem the person is facing. While the root cause of such problems is invariably located in the domain of demons and ancestral curses, the problems people face are usually of a highly sensitive and personal nature. The leader of the CIC is known to be interested in people's dreams and invites members of his congregation to meet him to interpret their dreams. This dream interpretation is never done in public but is a private affair for which seclusion is necessary.

These practices of deliverance are uniform to a large extent. Being slain in the Spirit is a component of a global Pentecostal discourse that has been extensively covered in books and magazines and on videocassettes which circulate widely in Pentecostal circles. The global discourse of deliverance is one of movement because it evidences how God and the heavenly powers provide for "breakthroughs" that "make a way" out of problematic situations and that unleash the power of the Spirit on the curses that keep people trapped in bondage to demons. This discourse of "loosening," of "untying," and of "breaking through" bespeaks the dichotomy of stasis versus movement, of seeking healing through movement as against the evil powers that keep the person trapped in troublesome circumstances. Although at first sight this discourse appears comparable to that of Maria ya Mvumbwe, it preempts the inquiry into the actual causes of being "stuck" that traditional healers would pursue through processes of divination because—and this is a crucial point—such inquiry into the depths of these forces may prove to be too dangerous. Inquisitiveness might enable the forces that require deliverance to entrap the leader and the healer. Why would any leader choose to put himself in such a dangerous position? Leaders and their helpers explained: "We are Africans, you see, we know the evil forces that our cultural traditions of demon worship tend to harbor, we need to expose them but we don't need to know too much of them. The Holy Spirit is ever more powerful anyway."

While deliverance is perceived as a universal panacea involving a highly uniform and standardized practice that makes it applicable to the healing practices in churches in the United States, Europe, and Africa alike, it is paramount that different cultural sources of evil be acknowledged. The praxis and discourse of deliverance recognize the situational nature of what evil is and how it is experienced but at the same time do not propound a situational or cultural understanding of its form, texture, or meaning. This praxis and discourse offers the possibility of a reformulation of a person's narrative by restating problems and solutions in a much more universal paradigm. It is not uncommon to hear about someone being delivered and about a "breakthrough" experience in Gaborone in much the same way as it would happen in Pentecostal churches in Ghana, Malawi, or the Netherlands (see van Dijk 1997).

Because these Pentecostal churches are transnational and their congregations often include members from a variety of ethnic and national groups, the churches are interested in addressing issues of identity as a path to healing social divisions. Also, in the current situation of Botswana, the churches are increasingly concerned with their members' recurrent problems relating to citizenship and "strangerhood."

Ethnic and national identity have become especially salient in Botswana, where government has stepped up its "localization policies" in recent years. These policies acknowledge the contribution foreign labor is making to the development of the country but favor local workers, even arguing that positions filled by non-Botswana should be handed over to local people. This is a reversal of the government's previous policies; after independence, Botswana recruited labor from various African countries to support government-related sectors such as education, health care, and the judiciary (Oucho 2000). In recent years however, xenophobic feelings have emerged as the local population has acquired the skills and qualifications necessary for these positions. Matters became further complicated by Botswana's unprecedented economic growth as a result of the discoveries and subsequent exploitation of diamond mines in the 1970s and 1980s (Jefferis 1998; Jefferis and Kelly 1999). This led not only to a growth in government expenditure and employment but also to an expansion of private enterprise in the country's rapidly emerging urban centers (Mosha 1998; Selolwane 2001).

Economic success and a growth in entrepreneurial opportunities contributed to more immigration, particularly from neighboring countries such as Zimbabwe, where the economic situation had deteriorated rapidly. It was in this context that the Botswana government began to strengthen the policies of localization it had introduced since Independence by tightening its immigration regulations and by engaging in a political debate concerning the rights and status of the society's minorities (see Werbner 2002a, 2002b; Nyamnjoh 2002; Selolwane 1998). Botswana's foreign workers have remained the prototypical eternal strangers. In the first decade after Independence it was clear that foreigners and expatriate labor posed no threat to the general objectives of creating a unified Tswana nation to which the Botswana government had committed itself. This is not to say that in the 1970s and 1980s no discussion ever erupted about the presence of foreigners in the country. This seemingly affirmed the success of the one-nation paradigm. As expatriates came to enjoy financial and other benefits or preferential treatment, there was little incentive for them to become citizens of Botswana. From time to time, public debates would focus on the benefits that foreigners were accruing, and these debates occasionally called for localization policies to ensure that jobs came into the hands of locals.

Over the last few years, such debates on the presence of foreigners and foreign labor have hardened and become more aggressive.[3] Both the public sphere and the media are becoming more and more xenophobic; Botswana seems more hostile to the presence of foreigners and the contribution foreign labor is making to the economy. Many foreigners who have become members of these new Pentecostal churches are now turning to leaders in the prayer-healing deliverance sessions with problems relating to their position in Botswana society. Their jobs are becoming increasingly insecure in sectors such as secretarial work, nursing, tailoring, and teaching, and there is a real danger that work and residence permits will not be extended because the government has decided that its own citizens should take over these positions. In a number of cases, the churches as a whole have come to be regarded as a *fremdkorper* and been criticized in the public domain as being "money-makers"—proponents of a religious ideology whose only goal is the exploitation of religion and religious convictions for the personal gain of its leaders.

Despite these social tensions and an increasingly negative public image associated with Pentecostal churches, the local population, particularly members of Gaborone's emerging middle classes, has become increasingly interested in joining these churches and, like the foreign members, appears to be highly attracted to the transnational image and transcultural practices the churches foster. Both the BLC and the CIC have established branches in other parts of the country and appoint local Batswana to their governing boards and ministries so as to appear fully localized. Both churches regularly discuss their responsibilities vis-à-vis personal healing, their moral position with regard to the nation, and, most important, the transnational composition of their membership.

However, while Pentecostal churches make every effort to downplay the significance of national identity by creating homogenizing rituals surrounding birth, death, marriage, and so forth, they cannot deny the Batswana public's feelings of uneasiness with the presence of foreigners and the increasing xenophobia being voiced in the media, where stronger views are expressed about the damage foreigners are causing the nation than those voiced by ordinary people in their day-to-day lives. Particularly in the CIC, concern over these issues has led to attempts to use religious means to heal the breach. Theirs can be called a form of social healing geared toward the a growing middle-class community of urban-based entrepreneurs and professionals who have an interest in superseding such divisions, for which the church provides an avenue.

Healing the Middle Class: Entrepreneurial Styles in a Foreign Country

While the CIC operates from Malawi and the international overseer of the church, a self-acclaimed bishop, resides in that country's city of Blantyre, Ghanaians lead the church in Botswana. The beginning of the church in Botswana was closely related to the spread of Ghanaian Pentecostalism (van Dijk 1997, 2001a, 2002a, 2003), which was tied to the massive emigration of Ghanaian labor that took place in the early 1980s and the subsequent establishment of Ghanaian diaspora communities in various parts of the world (Peil 1995; Manuh 1998; van Dijk 1997, 2001a). In the postcolonial development of Botswana, Ghanaians were recruited by the Botswana government to serve as teachers, university lecturers, hospital personnel, judges, and attorneys (see Otlhogile 1994), a program that started in the 1970s but gained momentum in later years. In the 1980s there were massive expulsions of Ghanaian labor migrants from Nigeria and an estimated 1.5 million Ghanaians were forced to look for employment elsewhere. Returning to their home country was no longer a viable option because of a sharp economic downturn and political instability. Botswana became an attractive alternative to migration to the West because of the prospects it offered for private enterprise in a booming economy. Ghanaians began establishing private businesses in places such as Gaborone and Francistown, an endeavor in which Ghanaian women in particular excelled (van Dijk 2002a, 2003). They became known for their hair salons and clothing boutiques and the colorful West African styles they successfully introduced to the Botswana public. Ghanaians became known in Botswana as an entrepreneurial class, and through their professions and businesses they established good relations with the emerging middle classes in urban Botswana society.

It was in this domain of middle-class entrepreneurialism that the new Pentecostal churches located many of their activities. In an ideological sense, prosperity and success are related to personal power and initiative, and Pentecostal leaders often operate as religious entrepreneurs, combining their spiritual zeal with private business; their ritual activities focus on the companies and businesses their members run. This element of Pentecostal ideology and ritual practice that caters to middle-class aspirations, hopes, and anxieties has been well documented for various parts of Africa and seems to have been prevalent in the way the Ghanaian-led Pentecostal churches in Gaborone attracted Ghanaian and other professionals and businesspeople. One explanation for this intertwined relationship between Pentecostalism and the middle classes is that members of this particular section of the population have a lot to gain but also a lot to lose and therefore face enormous uncertainties about their future socio-economic prospects, their public image, the way in which their status in society is influenced by public perceptions, and the way a discourse of modernity, which creates sharp divides between the "traditional" and the "modern," the inferior and the superior, the backward and the prestigious, works for them. Many feel uncomfortable being associated with "traditional" practices of healing and spiritual protection, however remotely, due to the ambiguities a discourse of modernity attributes to such activity. Yet they recognize that in the vagaries of the modern marketplace, the activities that constitute doing business still require spiritual care.

Therefore, Pentecostal leaders' services are much in demand and they offer spiritual healing and protection, such as ritual protection of shops and businesses against misfortune, attacks by rivals, and customer dissatisfaction. Pentecostal leaders in Gaborone make no secret of the fact that they visit members' shops and businesses to ritually cleanse and protect them against hazards. The modernist discourse of such services is one in which this activity is placed in juxtaposition to that of the "backward" and "ignorant" activities of traditional healers who do not rely on the "blood of Jesus" to make a business run smoothly but who use "relics" from a distant past that are already "demonic" because they use concoctions, potions, and herbs.

It is in this domain of ritual protection and strangerhood in a spiritual sense that the arrival of the Malawi-based but Ghanaian-led CIC became relevant. Starting in the early 1990s, Gaborone witnessed the arrival of a variety of Pentecostal churches from other parts of Africa that began to cater to the city's business community. The CIC, which operated simultaneously from Malawi and Ghana but trained and ordained its pastors in Malawi, was established in Botswana in 1994. From the start, it attracted many of the Ghanaian and other expat professionals in the city and members of the private business community. As I have described elsewhere (van Dijk 2003), dozens of Ghanaian salons, boutiques, and shops have opened in Gaborone over the last two decades, many of which fly in Ghanaian labor, mostly young girls, with the skills required to reproduce West African styles. But now Ghanaian owners have begun to employ more local labor due to localization policies. Many have been forced to look for understudies to manage their businesses in order to create opportunities for locals to take over eventually. These salons and boutiques have begun to serve as

places where Ghanaians and locals mingle. The shops have also begun to function as a training ground for Batswana hairdressers to learn the tricks of the
trade, to respond to and create specific styles, and to express a much more cosmopolitan style with regard to appearance and fashion than is common in
Gaborone. Now local women, and some men, use their employment in Ghanaian salons and boutiques as a period of apprenticeship when they can learn West
African styles as preparation for opening their own small businesses in the
future.

As a result, Ghanaian shops began experiencing increasing competition from
local salons in the 1990s and found themselves disadvantaged when the government decided to localize this business sector. After the late 1990s, Ghanaian
shop owners needed special permits to run hair salons and boutiques and were
required to obtain work permits for any workers they wanted to recruit in
Ghana. Even though the salons became a focal point for the government's localization policies, the general public still maintained a high level of fascination
with what the Ghanaians were able to offer.

Because they are a contact zone between locals and foreigners, the Ghanaian
shops and boutiques can also be seen as a kind of social compression chamber
where all sorts of moral values are exchanged. They are the places for the expression of identity and morality through the body, a location where all sorts
of exchanges take place in which perceptions of one's place in society, one's aspirations and ambitions are expressed and where a positioning vis-à-vis other,
perhaps less fortunate, groups in society is given shape and meaning. Also, the
shops allow the exchange of ideas concerning gender and generational roles in
society. These Ghanaian shops are usually owned by women in their late thirties
and early forties who have acquired a considerable level of socioeconomic independence through their businesses and who employ other and commonly
much younger hairdressers and tailors in their shops. This relative independence is ritually sanctified within the Pentecostal churches many of them belong to where the prevailing ideology in such churches maintains an image of
the man and the husband being the head of the family, thus prescribing a sub-
servient position to women and younger girls. While ideology and practice may
thus be contradictory, the shop owners would maintain that they engaged in
this business only after they had obtained the explicit consent of their husbands
and, in some cases also, some of the money needed to run the shop. Pentecostal
women who are shop owners capitalize on the modern ideology of the church
that positions the man as the head of the family by asking their husbands for
money to run their businesses; for them, this is a perfect symbiosis of the market
with Pentecostal ideology. Keeping the basic tenets of faith is a sure way to success and prosperity.

Hence, the construction of a shared morality is produced in the process of
shaping one's appearance according to what is fashionable and acceptable. Ghanaian shop owners are dependent on local customers and workers, and they
need to be acutely aware of how they and the businesses they run are perceived
in their eyes. They need to satisfy customer appetites and fulfill government

regulations with regard to the number of locals they employ, the opportunities they give for in-service training, and the taxes and fees they are supposed to pay. Local workers need to satisfy the demands of the customers as well as those of their Ghanaian employers and they have to understand how the Ghanaians perceive style, appearance, and beauty. The question then becomes how perceptions of the one in relation to the other are constructed in the triangle between shop owner, local worker, and customer and to what extent these are informed by preconceptions—perhaps even including xenophobic sentiments—of the Ghanaian owners and workers.

Local workers hardly ever make a career out of hairdressing itself. Hairdressing is mostly reserved for young Ghanaian girls flown into Botswana for that specific purpose. The local worker is commonly employed as the prototypical "shampoo girl," the one who touches the customer's skull in the first instance. Only after it has been washed will the Ghanaian hairdresser perform his or her magic tricks of transforming the hair and creating a new appearance. The shampoo girls form the first contact with the customer, the basic reason being the fear of HIV/AIDS and the Ghanaian preconceptions of local sexual morality. The general feeling among Ghanaian hairdressers is that they do not want to be the victims of what they perceive as an inferior sexual morality and be endangered through their work by contact with HIV.

This repulsion among Ghanaian hairdressers about working on unclean scalps is strengthened by another factor that increases their dependence on their local workers, putting them at the forefront of customer contact. From the Ghanaian perspective, hair is where spiritual powers can manifest themselves in the daily world. As hair grows from within the skull into an outer world, it is also an index for the mind and the spiritual powers located there. Ghanaian hairdressers are adamant that they will never do dreadlocks, as they are the ultimate sign of a demonic influence manifesting itself in the outward appearance of the person. While dreadlocks may be an extreme case, the relationship of hair with thought, spirit, and personal intentions makes doing hair a business for which additional spiritual strengthening and protection are required. Ghanaian hairdressers fear *muti*, and all the stories they hear make them generally feel at a loss as to where to locate *muti* with regard to its bodily manifestations. Local customers are suspected of bringing into the shop, perhaps unconsciously, certain powers that could destroy the business, the health, or the success a hairdresser enjoys. This is the second reason why the local shampoo girls are put at the forefront: the hope and expectation is that whatever the customer's hair may bring, it will affect them first. Ghanaian hairdressers expect shampoo girls to find their spiritual and protective *materia sacra* locally; most Ghanaian hairdressers feel such resources are not readily available to them.

It is in the domain of ritual protection and strangerhood in a spiritual sense that the arrival of the Ghanaian-led CIC became relevant. From the start, it adopted many of these salon and boutique owners and their expatriate workers. The church has become a haven for salon and boutique owners who are interested in spiritually addressing or redressing issues of nationality and localization. They feel the need to establish a close relationship with the leaders, and the church pastors regularly come and offer prayers and ritual sanctifications of the salons and boutiques, a kind of religious "sealing off" of external powers of affliction.[4] In addition, special prayers are held for all the staff working in a salon or boutique; these are gatherings the local workers are also expected to attend. These local workers have often not been exposed to Pentecostalism before and in talking to some of them it became clear that this was an encounter that only aggravated the experience of xenophobia they were confronted with.

One of the significant issues in terms of the feelings of superiority the Pentecostals tend to display in overcoming the "shortcomings of the nation and the ignorance of its citizens," as one of its leaders put it, is that these churches feel that they do better than the nation-state in providing the road to well-being of Botswana and reach out to include locals in their membership. Some of the hair salons have started to act as unofficial outstations for these churches; they help bring local workers and customers into contact with Pentecostalism or at least make them aware of its existence. First, when a nonbelieving local starts to visit a church because of one's actions and persuasive words, it is seen as a badge of one's faith in action. Doing the hair of a regular customer provides the time and the intimacy to discuss such matters on a regular basis. This builds on the concept that outward appearances may change someone into a new person; becoming born again adds an inside dimension to the process. Second, and perhaps even more important, building up long-standing relations with regular customers is vital for a salon or boutique's economic survival, particularly in view of increased competition from local owners. In addition, if clients become converted, this relationship will remain free of demonic influence—an influence that can have an adverse effect on the economic prospects of the business.

The awe and respect of locals for Ghanaian business and entrepreneurial acumen are strengthened by claims of the superior spiritual knowledge and power of these Pentecostal churches. These "claims to fame" work in tandem despite the fact that Pentecostal churches have been criticized in the public domain and the media. Foreigners are unpopular because they occupy jobs that should be in the hands of the local population and take business initiatives that leave fewer opportunities for the ordinary Batswana, and the churches are critiqued for being "money-making machines" that are foreign owned and fish in the ponds of the established churches for members.

Churches and salons are both acutely aware of the criticism leveled against them, which has led to questions in parliament about foreign influences in both hairdressing and church life.[5] It may thus be assumed that the interest churches and salons show in interacting with the local population is motivated by self-interest: the more interaction and commitment the less likely it is that localization will become any worse than it already is. Many Ghanaian actions, views, and ideas are inspired by notions of economic, spiritual, and even moral superiority, which may lead to the conclusion that their attitude is one of xenophobia. It is as if the way Ghanaians treat the shampoo girls and the way they perceive the girls' sexual morality as loose inform their sentiments of repulsion and leave no room for genuine fascination with forms of local social and cultural life. However, Pentecostal churches seem to play a role as places where marriages can be established with a kind of moral backing that they would otherwise lack. A number of Ghanaian migrants have married locally and have involved CIC church leaders as surrogate family marriage guardians responsible for negotiating the terms of the marriage on their behalf.

There appears to be an overabundance of border crossings of various kinds in present-day Botswana; a Malawian-based Pentecostal church under Ghanaian leadership is addressing issues of personal spiritual protection and national problems of a politics of identity. The church is stressing its multinational composition, its transnational way of operation, and its transcultural ritual repertoire; there is hardly anything typically Malawian about it. The Pentecostal identity is one that transcends national identities and is proclaimed capable of uniting its Ghanaian, Batswana, Zimbabwean, Malawian, and Kenyan membership by becoming part of a transnational community of confirmed believers. This ideology can be read as a form of cultural critique that proclaims to the general public that these churches do better in redressing xenophobia, contrary to government policies. While transnationalism may play a significant part in the operation of these churches, there is little in church teachings that refers to anything global in actual practice. Although the churches tap into globally circulating notions about religion and personal healing, these transnational features tend to respond to local circumstances. The perspective of globalization appears to offer little explanatory power where it comes to understanding why local people find the churches' boundary-crossing activities important in their daily affairs. This makes the postmodern experience of moving beyond the nation-state a process that is not a priori coterminous with globalization in the understanding of ordinary people. This form of Pentecostalism hardly makes a global space for imagination and practice for its confirmed believers, but it does make a transnational space where identities can be transcended so that one is not "stuck" within one nation. The geographical frame of reference remains largely regional in focus, although this regionality may extend from Botswana as far as Ghana and Nigeria. In that sense, this transnationalism in both its geographical and its symbolical frame of reference does not remain unbounded, as the term globalization in the field of Pentecostal studies usually tends to imply.

Conclusion and Interpretation: Elements of Regionality?

While they are becoming transnational in their focus and operation, Pentecostal churches are increasingly dealing with the nation and nationality as entities that create a need for healing and Christianization. While Pentecostalism's espousal of liberal ideology relates to the freedom of the individual, to liberties vis-à-vis family obligations, and to a fascination with middle-class entrepreneurial activity, it meets the nation-sate as a constraining factor. In the eyes of these churches, not only is the Botswana government's pursuit of liberalism and policies of localization contradictory, localization is also a cultural project that leaves no other option than to become "local" (in terms of identity and in terms of means of livelihood). In this sense, Ghanaians and their local counterparts feel that they become "stuck" in the nation-state; increasingly, the government's economic and political policies determine the scope of their activities, and the obligation to integrate into the local society is becoming harder to take. The Ghanaian entrepreneurial middle class is deeply motivated to engage in international relations as a profitable way of turning their businesses into successful ventures, and in a cultural sense they remain focused on transnational Ghanaian networks for exchanges that concern important events such as marriages and funerals. The churches transmit the notion that becoming "local" is a dead end, an avenue that does not lead to prosperity and exposure to a wider world, to their middle-class rank and file, no matter what national background they come from. In order to be successful in life, they tell them, their business and travels require that they be cut loose from whatever detrimental effects associated with nationhood they perceive. Pentecostalism provides a more suitable ideological framework for the middle classes in this context than other or earlier religious forms.

Regionality as a paradigm has been somewhat lost in the research on ritual practice and religious change in southern Africa. The 1970s and 1980s were marked by literature that explored religion in terms of its logics of place, its moral geography, and its symbolic and structural features of movement to and from important regional shrines, centers of healing, and other sacred places. This literature involved the regional study of territorial cults and explorations of the spread and local appropriation of certain healing practices and their socioreligious formations such as those including *ngoma* or those of the prophetic healing churches (see Janzen 1992; van Dijk et al. 2000a). The literature also focused on the study of ideological networks, the hierarchies of central places in shrine systems, the liminality of pilgrimage, and the relationship of all these manifestations of something inherently regional with processes of urbanization and long-distance labor migration. Crossing the precolonial/postcolonial divide, most of these studies demonstrate the wide-ranging significance of these religious forms in their capacity to connect localities and people over large distances, often beyond the boundaries of the post-independence nation-states. These connections, many argued, often existed in colonial and even precolonial times. Over time the significance of these forms of territorial cults, central shrines, and personal security cults increased because of the growth of labor migration. Labor migration from Malawi, or previously from colonial Nyasaland, mainly revolved around southern African mining and industry and thus was basically transnational more than it was rural-to-urban within the country itself. *Nyasas* ended up in the emerging industrial cities of South Africa, Zimbabwe, and Zambia or got stuck along the railway line leading from Johannesburg to Harare, forced to settle in places such as Francistown in Botswana. As a region marked by profound mobility both in geographical and social terms, religion played a significant ideological part in the settlement of migrants (see Spierenburg 2001 on the importance of spirit-mediums for the settlement of migrants in certain parts of Zimbabwe).

Prophetic healing churches became significant for creating a kind of ideological homecoming for the uprooted migrant in this context, and an extensive religious migration began to take place that spread these churches to various parts of the region. Improved methods of transport, in particular the colonial introduction of the bus (see Andersson 2001), allowed for easier and intriguing forms of long-distance consultation of *nganga* who had acquired region-wide reputations because of their healing powers. The activities of the famous healer B. Chisupe in Malawi (Probst 1999), who claimed to be able to cure AIDS through a new *mchape,* alluded to profound regional connotations by using the term, which as the early literature demonstrates, is related to its anti-witchcraft potential that bespoke the needs of people living in an area that covered parts of present-day Mozambique, Malawi, and Zambia and perhaps extending even to southern parts of Angola. Many came to visit him at his house near Zomba from far across the border.

My intention, however is not to rehearse the extensive literature about the many aspects of the relationship between the profoundly regional features of these religious formations and the people's perceptions of their fortunes in the processes of migration and mobility in this part of Africa. The question is instead the extent to which the new Pentecostal churches are building on these traditions of regionality, perhaps elaborating on them or critically engaging with them. The question of the regional character of these religious forms is important because recent studies, such as those on regional spirit possession in Behrend and Luig (1999) and those on the present-day significance of witchcraft in Moore and Sanders (2001), seem to place their discussions only in a modernist paradigm of the local versus the global. These authors investigate the way and the extent to which global modernities impinge on local religions and ritual practices directly. Little appears to be left of the explorations in an earlier literature of all the ways in which religious forms and rituals support the interconnection of localities in a wider but highly regionalized perspective. There is a tendency in the recent literature to present a bifurcated view in which local religious forms are examined for the ways in which they offer a particular understanding of the modern global world; a world which through modern means of communication and transport, through world economic systems and the modern media, is encroaching upon local societies and is interpreted as unsettling to local identities.

Going against the grain, I would argue that many of the religious forms I have discussed already espouse a sense of a wider world in their regional ways of operation and already mediate the local with that wider world determined by economic systems. As the boundaries of religious formations are never givens, they can emerge out of the politics of meaning, signification, and the subjective experiences of a sense of regionality (i.e., a sense of belonging to a particular region) in the confrontation with the wider world. Regionality in religious terms

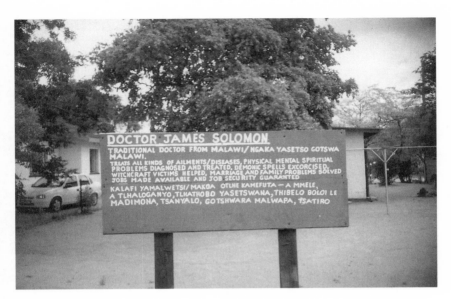

Photo by author.

presupposes at least ideological perceptions of connectivity between certain (and not all) localities on the one hand and a kind of critical distance with regard to the global on the other. Many of the prophetic healing churches, for instance the Apostolic churches such as those of the Masowe and Maranke Apostles, have become transnational by the sheer fact of their presence in a number of countries in this region but at the same time have remained distinctly regional in the sense that they have hardly branched out to other parts of Africa or beyond. Likewise, in the realm of traditional healing practices it is not difficult to see the importance local doctors attribute to being part of a regional system that enables them to attract patients and acquire their most potent medicines. In Gaborone, for example, many healers place signs along the roadside to let the public know that they are a "doctor from Malawi," even though most of them are not Malawian and did not do any medical training there. This identity mainly informs the general public that these doctors make the effort, on a regular basis, to travel to Malawi for certain roots, potions, and other materials that are in demand in Botswana. This connectivity in religious practice in the southern African region appears to have an essential element of empowerment. The substances and persons moving across borders and arriving from elsewhere in a locality in the region produce specific connotations of power: people see the substances arriving in Botswana from Malawi as undoubtedly the most powerful in their potential to both heal and harm.

Healing that comes from the outside creates high expectations about the powers involved, whether the border-crossing takes place when healers come from elsewhere or when clients visit a healer in another part of the region. As was the case with the *mchape* movements of the 1930s and 1940s in the region, which involved itinerant young men moving from place to place successfully eradicating witchcraft wherever they went, this potentiality is transcultural, transethnic, and, with the advent of postcoloniality, transnational in nature and involves a long history. In addition, and more important, this itinerant element in such religious practices would seem highly congruent with notions of the mobility of evil throughout the region. Witches are perceived as quintessentially mobile and their unseen nocturnal activities usually involve traveling large distances and crossing borders of any sort as they acquire new meanings in multiethnic and multicultural societies (Moore and Sanders 2001).

The most potent forms of evil have become increasingly regionalized to the extent that references to such concepts as *muti* can now be found in many societies in the region, even in places where the term did not exist before. Yet *muti* remains distinctly regional in signification; it does not resonate in other parts of Africa or beyond. In popular perceptions of this evil, witches use their *muti* to immobilize people, to paralyze them, to suck out their blood, to devour their meat and use human blood and bones to make airplanes with which to fly to South Africa and back again in an hour. People always describe the effects of witches' activities in their lives and social circumstances as the sense of being "stuck" and unable to move in a region where witches are active; the horizon of mobility is limited to the regional. It is, after all, primarily within the region that one finds employment, education, prosperity, healing and protection, and, last but not least, a spouse.

Although it is easy to point to certain factors that since historical times may have contributed to this regional horizon in religious affairs (extensive similarities in kinship, language, agricultural structures; a colonial history that fostered the idea of a political federation; a great degree of interdependence in terms of flows of trade, labor, and commodities), regionalism should not be conceived as something static. The features, meaning, and horizon of that regionality may become subject to change, as the rise of Pentecostalism in the region illustrates. In Botswana, there is a fascination with the powerful religious form of Pentecostalism that arrived from elsewhere. From the start it was clear to the general public that these churches were locating themselves in the heart of patterns of international migration in the region, which involves, among other things, the migration of labor to and from South Africa. They address and adopt the discourses on evil that are prevalent in society without becoming part of the localized forms of "syncretic" Christianity that are present in the hundreds of so-called candle churches, in which the burning of candles takes a central position in healing rituals in which a close relationship with vernacular forms and expressions of healing are important.

The two Pentecostal churches discussed here demonstrate in their practices how they are moving beyond the region and surpass the regionalized forms of interaction and exchange these syncretic churches depend upon. They add two dimensions of transnationalism that many of the other religious forms of healing lack. They transcend the nation-state by offering a transnational identity to their members. By becoming a confirmed believer one is born again into a new identity that qualifies being a national of a specific country, thus allowing for a perspective whereby the nation-state needs to be healed and its ills need to be treated. Pentecostalism addresses the crisis in the nation-state as it aims for a Christianization of the nation and a downplaying of national identities of the citizens *in* but not *of* a state (cf. Comaroffs). Obviously, this is particularly attractive for the transnational labor migrants who have moved from other African countries to Botswana and who form the majority of the membership of the two churches referred to here. Because of such mobility, Pentecostal churches such as the CIC play a role in the debates about xenophobia and display an interest in uniting foreigners and locals in their rank and file for political, social, and cultural reasons.

These churches are moving farther than the preexisting regional forms of healing in the transcultural ritual practices they organize that are neither local nor global. They emphasize a distinctly African cosmology in the forms of evil they acknowledge and contest. In this context, hair salons produce problems of xenophobia and illustrate the moral and spiritual dangers of evil powers related to beautification, seduction, and sexuality, the root causes of which lie in that specific cosmology. These are issues of protection and morality which are ultimately not perceived to be of a global nature but ones the churches understand they should fight in Ghana, Malawi, Botswana, and other parts of Africa. In addressing these ills by creating uniform ritual practices, there is ultimately no message for the "world"; the message is rather for the migrants of different African cultural backgrounds.

To conclude, the movement within Africa of churches and Pentecostal preachers and leaders has created a setting where Pentecostalism has become relevant in a context of transnational mobility in various parts of the continent. It is a context in which being "stuck" in one country may be experienced as an ill requiring treatment by a healer such as Maria ya Mvumbwe, involved as she is in wider regional systems of healing. Pentecostalism in Malawi and Botswana shows, however, that the meaning and significance of this regionality has become much wider than before, partly due to increased transnational migration and urbanization.

Notes

1. The parts of this chapter that deal with Botswana are from an earlier publication (Van Dijk 2003), for which permission was granted by *Africa* (journal of the International African Institute), which I hereby gratefully acknowledge.
2. The church recently claimed to have over 60,000 members spread throughout the 175 congregations in the country's twenty-four districts. It has opened ten branches in Mozambique and two in Tanzania.
3. Journalists seem to have a vested interest in discussing the issue of labor

immigration that has led to a stream of newspaper articles. One of the latest read: "Aliens Swamp Botswana. At Least One Illegal Immigrant Enters Botswana Every Three Hours. This Costs Botswana Pula 2,000 Every Hour" (*The Botswana Guardian*, August 9, 2002). Under the headline "Aliens Bashed: Parliament Attacks Foreigners," *The Botswana Guardian* (February 16, 2002) reported as follows on the Botswana Parliamentary discussions: "On Tuesday [February 13], Parliament underlined Botswana's hardening attitudes against foreigners with Francistown West MP Tshelang Masisi calling for a campaign to cleanse Botswana of undesirable expatriates. This has set off alarm bells among the expatriate community who feel the line between citizen empowerment and xenophobia has been blurred."

4. In Malawian Pentecostal churches, this practice is known as *kutsirika*, which has the connotation of keeping evil trapped and paralyzed at the doorstep. In Ghana, this practice is known as *nteho* and suggests ritual sanctification.

5. Although unemployment rates have been dropping (from 19.6 percent in 1998 to 16 percent in 2001), this is nevertheless a situation whereby even the predominance of Ghanaian-owned hair salons in the city has become a matter for parliamentary debate (*Mmegi Reporter*, June 2000).

6　From HIV/AIDS to *Ukimwi:*
Narrating Local Accounts of a Cure

Julian M. Murchison

One evening in 2000 in Peramiho, a town in southern Tanzania, I went to the home of friends for dinner. I was sitting in the courtyard area between the main house and the cooking area, visiting with Mama Asante as she prepared dinner.[1] She knew that my field assistant and I had been making regular trips to the local hospital to interview patients, and she asked if we had heard anything at the hospital about the woman that had given birth to a box. I had no idea what she was talking about and told her I had not heard anything about it. Knowing that the story was an intriguing one and probably suspecting that I would find it of particular interest, Mama Asante proceeded to recount the story for me:

> I heard the story yesterday from a woman who was visiting next door at my in-laws' house. This woman was an elderly woman from Mdundu-waro,[2] and she only spoke Kingoni. The Kingoni that she spoke was Kingoni of the interior. Even I didn't understand some of the Kingoni words that she was using.
>
> She told us about Neema,[3] a woman who lived near Mgazini.[4] Neema had gone through a regular pregnancy prior to giving birth, including going for regular checkups at the local clinic. When she went to the dispensary to give birth, she gave birth to a nice, clean wooden box! They opened up the box and inside they found a clean, new bottle labeled "*Dawa ya ukimwi*" ["AIDS medicine/cure"][5] in Kiswahili, but everything else was written in English, German, or some other language that they didn't understand.
>
> So they took it to the mission hospital in Peramiho for testing. But when they got to the hospital, the hospital staff told them they were unable to do that sort of testing there at the hospital in Peramiho, and they sent the bottle to Muhimbili[6] or somewhere like that for testing.

A night or two later, I was visiting the same friends in their sitting room. Mama Asante retold the story for her husband's sake since he had not heard it the first time she told it. Then she said there was an alternative version that she had heard recently at the water pump. Originally, an elderly man who lived down the road near the water pump told this version of the story, but Mama Asante had heard it retold among a group of women who had come to fetch water. A big crowd had gathered to listen. This version included some variations on the first version that Mama Asante told me and more details in a few respects.

Neema lived in the Mgazini area, had had a difficult life, and was in poor physical shape. She suffered from epilepsy. She even drooled on herself. And she was possessed by spirits. One day, these spirits came out and spoke. They acknowledged the suffering and hard life of their host. But they said they could not undo all the suffering and physical ailments. Instead, they were going to give her a gift in an attempt to offset those things. At that point, a nice bottle appeared on the table, with markings labeling it "*dawa ya ukimwi.*" First, she and the others who had gathered around her tried to pour some of it out into the bottle top to look at it, but it would not pour.

To demonstrate, Mama Asante motioned with her hands as if the medicine would pour halfway out and then retreat back into the bottle.

When they couldn't get the medicine to pour out of the bottle, Neema's family decided to take the bottle and the woman with her spirits to the hospital in Peramiho to see Dr. Ansgar.[7] When they arrived, Dr. Ansgar began to talk to this woman's spirits. The spirits explained to Dr. Ansgar that the medicine would only treat true AIDS patients and only required two spoonfuls. The spirits told him to bring a patient he was sure had AIDS. Dr. Ansgar sent for a patient, but when the patient arrived, the medicine would not pour. The spirits said, "This person doesn't really have AIDS. Bring us someone who does, one who has the symptoms, and you've tested." Dr. Ansgar sent for a second patient. The same thing happened, and the spirits repeated the same explanation. Finally, with the third patient Dr. Ansgar sent for, when they tried to pour the medicine, two spoonfuls came out, but not a drop more. This dose was administered to the patient, but nobody is sure what the status of things is. They don't want to call any attention to it until they have seen the results after three months.

Within a week, I heard several other versions of the narratives from different individuals. These stories about Neema and the *dawa ya ukimwi* generally laid out a relatively similar set of basic events but often differed in interesting ways in terms of the description and interpretation of the specific events. One narrator, who was obviously a bit skeptical, recounted this version for me:

Neema was a normal woman, not a traditional healer, not even a woman who knew some of the traditional medicine for children or anything like that. The only thing was that she had had spirits for an extended period of time. Then, one evening, her stomach began to bother her. At this point, she went to the bathroom only to find that she gave birth to a box. [Was she pregnant?] No, she wasn't pregnant.

So, she had this bottle, which didn't have a label or anything. Then her spirits came out and spoke for the first time, saying that this was *dawa ya ukimwi*. So Neema and her family brought it to Dr. Ansgar. He took it saying that it needed to be tested by experts, at which point the bottle disappeared. Because he was so excited about the possibilities, Dr. Ansgar was prepared to pay for Neema's food and other expenses for her to stay in Peramiho near the hospital, but she decided to return home.

When she arrived back home, the bottle reappeared there, and she began to treat people there. The bottle has a built-in *bao*.[8] In order to determine a patient's condition, she only has to pour the medicine into a spoon. If it will not pour, she knows this person does not really have *ukimwi*. Otherwise, the dose is two spoonfuls, and patients receive doses on a daily basis.

I asked if anybody had been cured yet, but they said they might know at the end of the week. They said they were still observing patients' outcomes. Still, I wanted to know if there had been any serious patients who had shown improvement. They told me that one woman from Mgazini or somewhere had been so critically ill at first that the first few days they had had to bring her by bicycle, but these days she was able to walk there under her own power.

Another interlocutor insisted that Neema had not given birth to the bottle or a box. Instead, this narrator focused on the role of Neema's spirits in the provision of the bottle:

Neema didn't give birth to the bottle and she wasn't pregnant. She did, however, have spirits that had bothered her for an extended period of time but had never spoken. She had even gone to see several traditional healers, who could not figure out what was wrong. One night she dreamed that all sorts of bottles were spread all over the place. Then, the next morning, she woke up and found a bottle on the pillow beside her. The bottle was the color of the palms of her hands.

When she woke up and found the bottle, she and her husband tried to figure out what it was and where it had come from. Then her spirits came out and spoke for the first time, revealing that it was *dawa ya ukimwi*. They took it to Dr. Ansgar, who was very excited, but when he went to try it on a patient, the bottle disappeared. It disappeared because the spirits had given certain restrictions, the chief one being that neither Neema nor the bottle should leave her home village. Patients should come to be treated there, and they should not be charged money.

The treatment is two spoonfuls, and it will not pour out if the person doesn't really have *ukimwi*. Plus, the medicine will never run out even though it is not a very big bottle. Dr. Ansgar is now taking *ukimwi* patients there to be treated, but they can't tell about the results because it hasn't yet been six months.

Analyzing and Interpreting These Narratives

In the middle months of 2000, I was living in southern Tanzania. I was engaged in a research project about the interconnections among traditional healing, biomedicine, and Christianity, and I became acutely aware that these stories were circulating about a local cure for AIDS. This story caught my attention for several reasons. First, several different people independently told me versions of the story that were very similar in terms of their form and content, though I think the differences between versions are also interesting and potentially illuminating. Second, in a condensed form, the story was remarkably illustrative of a number of important aspects of health and illness and HIV/AIDS in particular in southern Tanzania. Third, the story was a truly fantastic one and clearly captured the imaginations of the tellers of the story and my imagination as a listener.

Diseases and illnesses traverse and create boundaries in much the same way that healers, their medicines, and their practices do. This process has been particularly true in the course of the AIDS pandemic. In the narrative under consideration in this chapter, "AIDS" becomes "*ukimwi*" and occupies the landscape of southern Tanzania. However, the focus of this narrative and my accompanying analysis is not etiological or typological. The narrative begins with a presumed understanding about the sources and causes of illness. The focus is on treatment and a potential cure. The narrative involves humans, spirits, and a bottle of medicine traversing the local landscape in a series of compelling events that help to highlight the importance of particularly local understandings and experiences without forgetting larger-scale forces that influence these understandings and experiences.

The content of this particular story depends upon presumed boundaries that separate traditional healing and biomedicine, but the impetus for the story stems largely from crossing these boundaries by bringing elements and representatives of the two categories together. In the end, the boundary remains, but the story also provides a sense of the boundaries' permeability. This permeability may reflect the fact that despite the apparent clarity of the boundaries separating these conceptual categories, the practical concerns involved in the search for health lead many Tanzanians to cross and reshape these categories according to their own experience and needs. In southern Tanzania, traditional healing and biomedicine are both complementary and opposing categories. As such, they are mutually constitutive cultural categories; each one lacks meaning and context when separated from the other.

Stories about indigenous discoveries of AIDS cures or treatments in southern and eastern Africa are not uncommon (e.g., Probst 1999). *Ukimwi* is clearly a pressing health concern that affects Tanzanians, including residents of Peramiho and the surrounding area, both directly and indirectly. During the course of my research in 1999 and 2000, recurrent claims about a treatment or cure for *ukimwi* appeared in Tanzanian newspapers and in everyday conversations on a semi-regular basis; these claims are indicative of the search for an effective answer. Several traditional healers in the Peramiho area told me that they were hoping and seeking to identify medicines that would successfully treat *ukimwi*. In this context, these narratives about Neema and the *dawa ya ukimwi* become more intelligible. Responses to *ukimwi* have taken a variety of different forms, including the circulation of these narratives in the middle of 2000. Neema's story as an account of a cure is not unique or entirely new in general terms. However, the locally oriented specifics of the story merit attention as a window into local experiences with, and responses to, *ukimwi*.

Though I do not want to imply that these narratives are the conscious products of the narrators' pragmatic "agency," they are agentive in the sense that they represent significant degrees of semantic and symbolic control over *ukimwi* and associated concerns. In telling and retelling these stories, the narrators were firmly locating *ukimwi* on the local landscape and identifying local brokers and gatekeepers of power and authority. Thus, the narratives represent decidedly local responses to the HIV/AIDS pandemic that entail assertions of local control and power. In narration, these stories reflect upon and reshape multiple borders and boundaries. However, instead of closing these borders and boundaries, events and agents within the stories manage flows across these borders and serve to remap the local landscape and the borders in a way that allows the borders to be crossed without dissolving them. As a result of these narratives, the power dynamics associated with these borders shift and centers of power and authority are destabilized.

While these narratives represent a uniquely local response in many ways, they also fall into a larger category of responses to what Andersson has called "existential insecurity" (2002, 425). Andersson suggests that the presence of HIV/AIDS in Zimbabwe has contributed to a general situation of existential insecurity, but he is careful to clarify that HIV/AIDS is not the sole or even the primary reason for this situation of insecurity. The changing landscape of politics and economics has placed large amounts of stress on social structures and cultural systems (cf. Ashforth 2002). When we extend this notion of insecurity to other parts of southern and eastern Africa, we encounter numerous different responses (see, for example, Yamba 1997 and Mogensen 1997).

In a case that in many ways bears striking similarity to the narratives about Neema and the *dawa ya ukimwi*, Probst describes *mchape '95*, during which large numbers of people in Malawi traveled to the southern part of the country to drink a medicine that was supposed to cure AIDS. Chisupe, the healer responsible for this medicine, discovered it as a result of directions he received in a dream. Directions in a subsequent dream informed him of the proper dose, that he was not supposed to charge for the medicine, and that he was not to take the medicine elsewhere. These events and the large numbers of people who traveled to see Chisupe garnered the attention of the national media and the Malawian government. While Chisupe and the movement were subject to some government scrutiny and contestation, Probst does not want to reduce *mchape* '95 to oppositional resistance in terms of Chisupe against the state. Instead, he argues that Chisupe provides an intriguing counter to the power of the state and "biopower" without direct confrontation and resistance. Probst is most concerned with public negotiations and discourses as knowledge of Chisupe spread across the country and people traveled great distances to visit him. For Probst, *mchape* '95 was a fleeting historical moment that served as a "cleansing of the nation" in post-Banda Malawi (Probst 1999, 134).

The narratives about Neema and the *dawa ya ukimwi* never produced national attention or large groups of people journeying in search of treatment. Therefore, I will not interpret these narratives on a national scale in the same way that Probst does for *mchape* '95. The number of different occasions on which I heard these narratives clearly indicated that the stories had entered the local public imagination, and I want to place and analyze the narratives in the context of that specifically local imagination. The parallels between Chisupe's and Neema's stories remain interesting and may have similar symbolic relevance, but the differences in the stories come into relief when examined from a local perspective.

In the analysis that follows, I seek to examine the narratives carefully as forms of knowledge that do not necessarily make sense within scientific or rationalist epistemologies. Opening scholarship to the possibility of other epistemological standpoints has meant opening up to the possibilities of alternative forms of knowledge (e.g., Nyamnjoh 2001). Narratives, particularly those that appear fantastic or fictional from an outsider's perspective, represent one such form of knowledge. Recent Africanist scholarship has turned to narratives about cannibalism, vampires, trade in human skins, witchcraft, and ritual murder as important sources to be analyzed from both historical and anthropological perspectives (cf. White 1995, 1997, 2000; Burke 2000; Sanders 2001; Bastian 2001; Comaroff and Comaroff 1993, 1999; Pels 1999; Musambachime 1988).

Stories involving supernatural elements and other seemingly fantastic aspects are not uncommon in contemporary Tanzania. In 1999, stories about skin harvesting captured the nation's public imagination (see Sanders 2001). During my research in and around Peramiho, at least one neighboring village received a series of public notices alleging the use of witchcraft to harm and kill the youth in the village. These notices merited enough attention to call a public meeting of the local government with the residents of the village. These types of stories and their ability to captivate Tanzanians' imaginations to one degree or another often make sense as commentaries, albeit fragmentary and indirect, on local and national experiences with the global political economy (see Sanders 2001). In much the same way, the stories about Neema serve as commentaries on local experiences with the HIV/AIDS pandemic and biomedicine, including some reference to the role of the global political economy.

Luise White's *Speaking with Vampires* (2000) represents one of the richest and most comprehensive considerations of how to analyze these forms of storytelling and narratives as forms of knowledge and sources of information. White suggests that the single most important premise of her analysis is that

> people do not speak with truth, with a concept of the accurate description of what they saw, to say what they mean, but they construct and repeat stories that carry the values and meanings that most forcibly get their points across. People do not always speak from experience—even when that is considered the most accurate kind of information—but speak with stories that circulate to explain what happened. (White 2000, 30)

She follows this statement by clarifying that she is not suggesting that people intentionally tell false stories (see Ellis 1993). From this perspective, the act of narration is history. How the story is told is at least as important as the factual content.

White is careful to point out the problematic nature of terminology such as rumor and gossip to refer to stories that narrators assume to be true. Still, given these terminological shortcomings, she builds a compelling argument for engaging the narratives of rumor and gossip analytically. Both White and Peter Pels have analyzed rumors about vampires in colonial Africa as important historical sources about local experiences and perceptions. In his treatment of these rumors, Pels asserts that rumors about white vampires in colonial Tanganyika have metaphorical significance as a reflection of indigenous Tanganyikans' experiences with different forms of colonial contact (Pels 1999). In my analysis of the narratives about Neema and the *dawa ya ukimwi*, I suggest that many aspects of these narratives have similar metaphorical significance. However, I am unwilling to offer a single interpretation of these narratives. As White points out, the "diverse and contradictory elements" (85) of rumor contribute to the richness and complexity of these narratives: "Asking, let alone deciphering, what a rumor is about makes a rumor about one thing. It makes rich texts of half truths and local knowledges linear and simplified" (83).

From this perspective, seemingly contradictory or fantastic claims (such as giving birth to a box) do not represent stumbling blocks for analysis. Spirits' conversations with Dr. Ansgar and the disappearance and reappearance of the bottle become the building blocks for analysis. The sort of analysis that I propose, however, is not premised on building a grand structure in the end. Instead, I aim to engage with that spirit of playfulness and irony that Mbembe has argued is part of the "banality of power" in postcolonial Africa (Mbembe 1992; see also van Dijk 2001b). On these terms, the narratives engage and address issues and figures of power, but they do so indirectly and often playfully. We can identify elements of resistance, but these instances represent something more than simple resistance to powerful structures and institutions. In this playful, fantastic, and slippery form, the result is not direct confrontation or upheaval, but rather a reconfiguring of perspective that privileges local epistemologies.

Biomedicine, Dr. Ansgar, and the HIV Test

When I first heard the story from Mama Asante, the vivid imagery of the box and bottle and the dramatic act of the woman giving birth grabbed my attention, but I found the accounts of the events in Dr. Ansgar's office at the hospital equally remarkable. As the medical superintendent of the mission hospital, Dr. Ansgar was a widely recognized symbol of the hospital and its administration. Plus, as both a European doctor and a Benedictine monk in residence at the adjacent abbey, he served as a representative figure of both biomedicine and Roman Catholicism, the predominant religion on the local landscape. Due both to his public recognition and to his relatively unique role as a permanent European doctor,[9] visitors to the hospital occasionally sought out Dr. Ansgar specifically for consultation and treatment. In the eyes of at least some Tanzanians, his identity as a white European linked him more closely and directly to biomedicine than even his well-qualified and incredibly able Tanzanian colleagues. From a formal interview and informal conversations with Dr. Ansgar, I knew that he was highly skeptical of many of the treatment claims of traditional healers in the area and that he was particularly skeptical about claims of spirit possession and witchcraft. Therefore, the detailed account of the interaction between Neema's spirits and Dr. Ansgar in his office, which appears in several versions of the story that I heard, struck me as highly ironic and illustrative.

Science and biomedicine are part of the contemporary lives of most Tanzanians and other Africans, even if they have only partial knowledge of, or access to, them. The presence of various forms of science and biomedicine does not mean that other cultural forms have disappeared. Therefore, as Andersson (2002) suggests, talking about the clash of biomedical and traditional epistemologies is disingenuous. As they face these circumstances, Tanzanians and others do not simply make a choice between alternative ideologies or exchange one ideology for another. They shape and construct their own understandings and sets of knowledge about treatment options and illnesses, including *ukimwi*. From a perspective concerned with the social production of knowledge, the ideas and conversations that emerge locally serve as important alternative forms of knowledge about HIV/AIDS. The narratives about Neema and other locally emergent forms of knowledge serve to evaluate and reshape questions of power, authority, and efficacy. Here, biomedicine does not disappear, but the flows between biomedicine and traditional healing (and other pertinent categories, as we shall see) are local phenomena subject in large part to local control.

The story and this sequence of events in Dr. Ansgar's office effectively call into question science's perceived infallibility and the claims of biomedical personnel that they are the only legitimate, or at least most effective, healers in the area.[10] Here, the question of agency becomes an essential one. In the story, Dr. Ansgar emerges as an ineffectual and even possibly deceitful agent in the treatment of *ukimwi*. At the same time, the spirits—to whom Dr. Ansgar and others would deny an existence—are effective agents able to act in a situation where Dr. Ansgar is unable to do so. They are able even to correct any mistakes that Dr. Ansgar and the rest of the hospital staff may have made in terms of diagnosis.

In light of biomedicine's relative ineffectiveness in treating, and especially in curing, HIV/AIDS in the local context (and in Sub-Saharan Africa generally), this story offers a potential alternative for the source of treatment and cure. At its most transparent surface level, the story seems to reassert the efficacy of treatments rooted in traditional healing directly in the face of biomedical treatment. It also holds out the possibility of misdiagnosis at the hospital. As a whole, the story undermines the sense of biomedicine, embodied in the figure of Dr. Ansgar, as therapeutically and socially omnipotent. The story shows that biomedicine is occasionally mistaken and relatively impotent in the face of *ukimwi*. The seat of therapeutic efficacy in this case lies some fifteen to twenty miles away in Mgazini.

As tools of the different agents involved in the accounts, different forms of testing become emblematic of the abilities and limitations of these agents. The scientific HIV test emerges as fallible and/or unimportant. Given the lack of any tangible results from a positive HIV test and the general reluctance on the part of all parties to engage in testing, the depiction of the HIV test as unimportant is not surprising.

In this context, the *bao* connected to the bottle and the spirits' supervision of its use offers an alternative means of testing, one that presumably is less fallible and more effective. This effectiveness is in fact directly linked to the mechanism of the *bao* itself. If the *bao* reveals the patient to have *ukimwi* by allowing the *dawa* to pour into the spoon, then the medicine is ready for administering to the patient. In stark contrast to the biomedical hospital's inability to offer treatment following a positive test, the *bao* leads directly into treatment.

This superficial reading and interpretation of the story in terms of biomedicine's limitations and potential fallibility only scratches the surface in terms of examining the key issues and themes associated with health and illness and the local landscape. Delving deeper into this story and its emergent themes and imagery allows us to examine physical and conceptual boundaries. This story depends on several different sets of boundaries that are crucial to the sequencing of events and that ultimately make the story a compelling form of social knowledge.

Traditional Healing and Biomedicine

The first boundary between traditional healing and biomedicine becomes clear as soon as Neema and her companions arrive at the hospital in Peramiho to meet with Dr. Ansgar. In contrast with Dr. Ansgar, the possessing spirits represent the opposing category of traditional healing. Biomedicine is generally ineffective in treating conditions associated with spirit possession; traditional healing, on the other hand, is the most effective form of treatment for these conditions. In some cases, spirits explicitly reject biomedical treatment by refusing to allow their hosts to receive injections at the hospital.

In this story, Neema, her spirits, and the bottle containing the *dawa* cross this boundary to visit Dr. Ansgar but ultimately end up recrossing the boundary in their return home. The acts of crossing and recrossing are both significant acts in the course of the story. Exemplified by the movements associated with crossing and recrossing these boundaries, the conceptual categories of traditional healing and biomedicine are overlaid on the local landscape in the course of the narratives.

The Local Landscape

Mama Asante and others who told me the story generally all began by explaining that Neema, the woman in question, resided in Mgazini. Mgazini was a village about twenty miles from Peramiho, and local residents frequently made trips back and forth between the areas, but residential and public life differed greatly between the village and Peramiho. Neema's residence in Mgazini meant that she lived in a less accessible rural location than the residents of Peramiho who were telling me the story. In the area, there were significant differences in the role of the cash economy and the availability of transportation from one community to another, and Mgazini clearly represented a more rural, more "traditional" village lifestyle. In this context, Peramiho represented a more "modern" location, marked by the presence of the Benedictine abbey with its hospital and other influential social institutions as well as two large markets and access to Songea, the regional seat of government and largest urban area in the region.

In much the same way that the story involves crossing the conceptual boundaries between traditional healing and biomedicine, the trip from Neema's home in Mgazini to the hospital in Peramiho (and back again) involves crossing the boundary between the village and Peramiho. Occasionally the local government would set up gates along the roads from these villages to Peramiho to prevent the transport of harvested crops and other goods without the payment of the proper taxes. However, these occasional physical boundaries were only temporary and less important than the boundary between the two spheres marked by differences in clothing, language, and economic resources, among other things. Neema's association with Mgazini places her in the heart of a cluster of symbols and ideas that links rural village life to nature and the root or heart of tradition. These symbols and ideas often represent the source of power and validity for traditional healing. Neema as the source of the bottle and medicine at the heart of the story is firmly rooted in this symbolic nexus in the way each person began telling me the story, but the story involves both her and the bottle crossing the boundary between Mgazini and Peramiho.

Linguistic Boundaries

Linguistic differences and barriers are a third recurrent theme in the story. The first time I heard this story, Mama Asante began by remarking on how she had heard the story from an elderly woman who only spoke Kingoni.[11] Mama Asante made a point of saying that the woman spoke Kingoni from the interior to the point where she had used words with which Mama Asante, a fluent Kingoni speaker, was unfamiliar. Kingoni was widely spoken in many contexts in Peramiho. However, Kiswahili, the national language, was the most widely spoken language in the multiethnic community of Peramiho, particularly in public spaces.

The story's origin in the person of a Kingoni speaker indexed its geographic origin in the more rural area of Mgazini or at least the intermediate village of Mdunduwaro. The way that Mama Asante proceeds to tell the story allows the listener to project the original narrator's use of Kingoni onto Neema. Mama Asante's reference to the narrator's use of "Kingoni of the interior" is notable in this respect. The use of Kingoni is consistent with her location in Mgazini and again indexes a more "traditional" perspective.

The narrator's use of Kingoni stands in stark contrast to the appearance of words in English or some other European language such as German on the bottle in Mama Asante's version of the story. The appearance of these words below the Kiswahili phrase "Dawa ya ukimwi" is intriguing. Kiswahili is the language of primary education in Tanzania and is widely spoken. English, on the other hand, is the language of secondary- and university-level education, and proficiency in English generally serves as a strong practical indicator of education and social prestige. In the story, the Kiswahili phrase on the bottle allows the people involved to identify readily the basic purpose of the bottle and its contents, but questions raised by the words in English or German prompt them to travel to Peramiho to seek out Dr. Ansgar. In this version, the foreign words on the label of the bottle index scientific biomedicine. These words effectively point the way to the hospital.

Knowledge and Testing

The story does not simply ignore or abdicate any role for biomedicine. Instead, Neema and her companions, both human and spiritual, seek out biomedical validation without relinquishing control. Dr. Ansgar and Muhimbili represent arbiters of biomedical knowledge. In some sense, they serve as gatekeepers of this knowledge. But the same bottle that prompted Neema and her companions to seek out these gatekeepers ultimately evades their control.

The end of each of the different versions of the story is seemingly anticlimactic. The implication is that the *dawa* will help patients, but the time lag and the nature of *ukimwi*'s manifestations make confirmation of that improvement impossible. Still, even without definitive resolution, the story remains compelling, largely because of its ambiguity, particularly concerning the role of biomedicine.

The issue of scientific testing emerges when the bottle is taken to Dr. Ansgar for testing or people discuss the possibility of sending it to Muhimbili. In these locations, personnel will presumably run tests designed to determine the chemical and pharmacological properties of the *dawa* in the bottle. Nobody ever addresses the question of how they are going to run tests on the *dawa* if they cannot pour it out of the bottle, but here a general confidence in scientific testing seems to reemerge in the course of the story. Indeed, the people who told the story to me seemed to imply that sending the bottle for tests was a logical step in terms of following through on the *dawa*'s effectiveness. Nevertheless, in at least two versions of the story, the bottle disappears before any such tests can be undertaken. Perhaps this disappearance indicates the general incompatibility of these approaches. After all, the *bao* has already demonstrated the inappropriateness of biomedicine's HIV testing. Submitting the *dawa* to scientific testing would seem to do little more than offer a chance for science and biomedical personnel to appropriate this medicine and technology for themselves. This sort of appropriation would be an improper response to such a local solution, and the bottle's disappearance means that such a response is impossible. In this scenario, the practical evidence of whether a patient's condition improves will be the principle indicator of the *dawa*'s effectiveness.

While each version of this story focuses decidedly on the local level and on boundaries operating at the local level, the story also hints at boundaries operating on other levels. References to Muhimbili, the use of English, and the figure of Dr. Ansgar, a European monk, are all important in this regard. Each of these references indexes national and international scales of reference and the associated boundaries (i.e., Peramiho/Dar es Salaam; Swahili/English; Africa/Europe; North/South). Muhimbili, the English language, and Dr. Ansgar as symbols all point away from Peramiho and the immediate surrounding area. Since they each represent forms of scientific knowledge, their indexical relationship to geographically removed locations (principally Dar es Salaam and Europe) is revealing in terms of how this story as a locally produced form of knowledge relates to scientific constructions of knowledge that claim to be universal. Each of these symbols remains important and powerful in its own right, but its direct power and influence is fragmentary as a result of the events in the narratives.

Local Power Brokers and Gatekeepers

As Luedke and West point out in the introduction to this volume, many traditional healers in southeast Africa gain validity and power by crossing boundaries and physically traversing the landscape. In some ways, this crossing of boundaries is as true of biomedical doctors as it is of traditional healers. In Peramiho, people seek out Dr. Ansgar because he is from Germany, and many of the most respected doctors at the hospital are from other parts of Tanzania. Several have traveled internationally to study. Similarly, in Peramiho, many of the most successful and popular traditional healers come from geographically distant places such as Mbamba Bay, Sumbawanga, Malawi, and Mozambique. In some cases, their migration to Peramiho involved crossing national borders. Healers who are longtime residents of the area generally are accorded less authority and power by residents. Patients also frequently travel long distances to seek out specific healers in specific locations.

In contrast with these foreign sources of healing power and authority, the primary source of power and authority in this case appears to be decidedly local. The story chronicles the local origin of a treatment for *ukimwi*. The source of power and authority in this story does not seem to come primarily from the crossing of regional or national boundaries. Instead, the source of power and authority resides in or emerges from within the person of Neema, a female resident of Mgazini. Some cynical interpretations of the story suggested that Neema was spreading a rumor designed to ensure her success as a healer claiming to treat *ukimwi,* but I never heard of her subsequent emergence as a healer. From a less cynical perspective, she appears to be a reluctant or surprised participant. She has suffered with spirit possession and other maladies according to several versions of the story, but she will remain a suffering patient. The story does not involve her crossing the boundary between suffering patient and healer. In many ways, she is a nonvolitional agent for the delivery of this *dawa ya ukimwi.* She does not speak. The primary volitional agents appear to be the spirits that possess her. These spirits exude power and authority and serve as the primary border-crossers and border guards in the course of the story. Only after they emerge and begin to speak are Neema, her relatives, and others fully aware of what has transpired.

The spirits' power and authority is at no point more apparent than when they command an audience with Dr. Ansgar in his office at the hospital. The narrators of the story were almost certainly aware that only the most unusual of circumstances would prompt Dr. Ansgar to entertain what he would surely consider to be a fanciful story. A potential AIDS cure presumably qualifies as the most unusual of circumstances. Not only does Dr. Ansgar entertain and converse with Neema's spirits in his office, but the spirits seem to question Dr. Ansgar and give him orders. Because they possess and control the bottle containing *dawa ya ukimwi,* they are in control. They cross the boundary into the hospital and the realm of biomedicine and take charge. The spirits establish the conditions for the administration of the medicine, and the built-in diagnostic mechanism reinforces their control over its administration as Dr. Ansgar provides patients for testing. In at least one version of the story, the spirits required that the *dawa* be used only in Neema's home village.

Because the power of and over the bottle of *dawa ya ukimwi* lies with the spirits, this treatment cannot be replicated or appropriated by others. It is local in origin and the spirits will administer and control it locally. In this story, one can see that the spirits as supernatural agents construct a sort of boundary around their medicine and their knowledge. This boundary is crucial. In a time when local forms and local knowledge are often purchased or appropriated as part of the process of commodification, this particular item cannot be appropriated and commodified through scientific means. This resistance to appropriation implicitly calls into question common assumptions that any efficacy traditional healing enjoys can be reduced to an almost protoscientific knowledge of herbal medicines that modern scientific testing can confirm and refine. Instead, this knowledge takes a decidedly different form that cannot be subsumed under science or biomedicine. Dr. Ansgar and the others in the story want to submit the bottle for testing. Even the spirits seek the validation that would come with successful treatment of patients under Dr. Ansgar's supervision at the hospital. However, the spirits' words and the bottle's physical disappearance and reappearance suggest that the boundaries protecting local control of this form of knowledge are more important. Neema, her spirits, and the *dawa ya ukimwi* all return to her home village and are firmly embedded in the symbolic framework of local knowledge.

Power and Politics

According to Brooke G. Schoepf, "Response to AIDS is political everywhere. Knowledge is socially situated, built on previous knowledges with the power to define how we know" (2001, 338). In this general sense, the narratives about Neema and the *dawa ya ukimwi* are political instances of contestation, providing a counter to hegemonic knowledge claims. Though the primary focus of these narratives is illness and treatment rather than government political structures, they are political in much the same way that Ellis (1993) suggests *radio trottoir* ("pavement radio"; the informal discussion of current affairs common in urban areas) is a popular political form in Togo. However, these narratives are not emblematic moments of a grand resistance movement. They obliquely and playfully engage figures and symbols of biomedicine and aspects of the global political economy. Both the narrators and the listeners (including myself) seemed to delight in their semantic ambiguity and irony. In many ways, these attributes are the source of the narratives' greatest power.

The currency of these narratives and their apparent wide circulation among residents of the area indicate that the stories had entered the imagination of many members of the community. As such, the story resonated with a number of important themes and issues concerning health and illness in the area. Experiences involving *ukimwi*, as with other illnesses, are interconnected with social institutions and with cultural symbols and practices, and the stories are emblematic of these intricate connections. The narratives engage and shape local politics as they include, address, and question influential nodes of power, most notably in the figure of Dr. Ansgar and the mission hospital and through more oblique references to national and international sites of power and authority. At the same time, the narration of these stories constitutes local figures, symbols, and seats of power that reside in (and traverse) the local landscape. In the course of the narratives, these local figures become the primary brokers and gatekeepers of knowledge and power.

These narratives stand in stark contrast to scientific and biomedical narratives about HIV/AIDS. In many ways, practitioners of scientific biomedicine produce and disseminate a potentially hegemonic body of knowledge about HIV/AIDS, specifically about means of infection, the course of the disease, and hopes for treatment or a cure. The stories of Neema and the bottle containing *dawa ya ukimwi* offer alternative ways of seeing and knowing that seem to be counterhegemonic even if they do not easily fall into the category of resistance.

The story of HIV/AIDS in the area is not a straightforward one encapsulated in a scientific or biomedical version. Instead, the stories that involve spirits and seemingly magical elements offer a different perspective on experiences with *ukimwi*. As forms and representations of local forms of knowledge, they call into question the dominant scientific and biomedical narratives about HIV/AIDS, but, more important, they start from an entirely different epistemological stance and represent an incomparable if not incongruous form of knowledge (Barbour and Huby 1998; Schoepf 2001).

Ukimwi and Related Health Concerns

As a local form of knowledge, this story is not simply an isolated flight of fantasy, even if some of the events in various versions of the story seem fantastic, particularly to outsiders. In other narratives produced by outsiders about Sub-Saharan Africa, HIV/AIDS often becomes representative of the general health of African individuals and groups and appears to exist in a context devoid of others illnesses and concerns. This narrative, in contrast, indirectly connects experiences with *ukimwi* to other important health concerns on the local level. My own research clearly demonstrated that spirit possession, fertility, and epilepsy/convulsions were all very important health issues in and around Peramiho, and different versions of the story referenced each of these issues. Neema, the woman at the center of the narrative, embodies all three of these central health concerns. Consequently, *ukimwi* is not the only health concern in the story; it appears as one of a number of local interconnected health concerns, which include spirit possession, fertility problems, and epilepsy.

In the Peramiho area, spirit possession was a relatively common health concern, particularly among women. Neema will presumably remain the host for these spirits. As this story demonstrates, spirit possession can have both positive and negative results. The nature of these results depends largely on the extent to which the human host and spirits are able to develop a relationship that allows them to coexist. Clearly the spirits in this case are acting positively by providing the *dawa* for treatment of *ukimwi,* but in all likelihood their host will continue to live as a suffering patient. Because this story brings together spirit possession and *ukimwi,* we begin to see that perhaps *ukimwi* is not an entirely separate or overpowering health concern. It relates to a number of other health issues that confront local residents.

Difficulties with fertility represent another set of health concerns in the narrative. Because *ukimwi* raises concerns about fertility, it is a particularly pressing health concern both for the individual and society generally (see Setel 1999). With that in mind, the fact that Neema *gives birth* to the *dawa* in several versions of the story appears almost poetically significant. Presumably this *dawa* will allow recipients to give birth to children who are free of the risks and problems associated with *ukimwi*. In this seemingly fantastic act of Neema giving birth to the box or the bottle, the story reflects the important ties between fertility/childbirth and *ukimwi* as primary health concerns.

More generally, that Neema gives birth to the box seems to index women's procreative and generative powers. Despite male dominance in many publicly recognized areas in southern Tanzania, women are active performers and producers of cultural realities, particularly as they relate to experiences of health and illness. Because of cultural expectations about caregiving and domestic responsibilities, many of the social and economic burdens of *ukimwi* have fallen on women. In addition, the relative risk of infection for men and women means that women are increasingly overrepresented among those infected and therefore subject to the direct physical burdens of the illness. Here, Neema embodies the generative power to cure *ukimwi* and to reduce those burdens. Women are not dependent on the largely male-dominated field of biomedicine for a cure or an answer.[12]

In Mama Asante's version of the story, Neema also suffers from epilepsy, a third important health concern. Epilepsy (*kifafa*) is another polyvalent illness in southern Tanzania marked by existential uncertainties. In attempts to manage their condition, patients frequently make use of diagnosis and treatment from both traditional healing and biomedicine. In some cases, epilepsy connects directly with experiences of spirit possession. Therefore, Neema's own experiences with epilepsy link her and her story to the larger complex of local health concerns.

By linking these other health issues to *ukimwi*, the telling of the story reflects the fact that *ukimwi* is a central health concern, but not one that eclipses or is separate from other health concerns. These other concerns do not disappear in the face of *ukimwi*, despite the intense focus on HIV/AIDS on the national and international levels in particular. As Neema, her spirits, and the bottle travel across the local landscape in the story, *ukimwi* emerges as a locally salient illness but also one that is part of a larger spectrum of local health concerns and subject to some degree of local control.

In offering this retelling and interpretation of this story, I am not suggesting that biomedical knowledge about HIV/AIDS is unimportant. Nor do I think that the original narrators from whom I heard these stories would take that position. HIV/AIDS is a very important health concern globally and needs attention from the spheres of both biomedicine and political economy. The Tanzanians who told me these stories narrativized their knowledge and experiences in a fundamentally different way from the dominant biomedical narrative about HIV/AIDS; in doing so, they crossed a sort of boundary between HIV/AIDS and *ukimwi*. On one level, *ukimwi* and HIV/AIDS are the same. Everyone involved would probably agree on means of transmission, symptoms, and the suffering involved. However, *ukimwi* indexes different boundaries and enables different agents, particularly in the course of these narratives. These narratives seem to reflect some degree of frustration with biomedicine's ineffectiveness in the face of *ukimwi* on a local level, but, more fundamentally, the narratives reflect a form of local political power rooted in semantic and symbolic control of boundaries and the flows across these boundaries. In narrating these accounts about *dawa ya ukimwi*, residents of Peramiho were asserting control in a context in which they often lacked control over many aspects of their lives and their health. Neema, a woman from Mgazini, gives birth to the box. Her spirits refuse to allow the bottle to be sent for testing. The *dawa ya ukimwi* originates at the local level, and the controlling agents remain there as gatekeepers and brokers.

In telling and retelling these stories, the narrators are making and shaping history and culture in the face of suffering and uncertainty. These stories and their narrators effectively manage the physical and categorical boundaries that emerge as relevant in relationship to *ukimwi*. In the course of the stories and their narration, the spirits and the storytellers become important brokers and gatekeepers of knowledge and boundaries on the local level. The end result is a powerful set of narratives that serves to redraw both physical and conceptual boundaries and to manage flows across these boundaries.

HIV/AIDS does not simply invade the local landscape and assert its control over it. *Ukimwi* is nested within a complex system of flows and stops managed at the local level. These narratives are captivating examples of local responses to existential insecurity that exemplify the resilience of humans and the role of cultural creativity in contexts of suffering and uncertainty. They serve as a powerful reminder that even in the face of a global pandemic, local actors and agents play a powerful role in mapping and managing borders and boundaries.

Notes

This research was conducted under a research permit granted by the Tanzanian Commission for Science and Technology (COSTECH) from 1999 to 2000. I wish to thank them and all the other Tanzanians who were gracious hosts and made this research and this chapter possible. Millsaps College and the Hearin Foundation provided support for the writing process. In the course of that process, Tracy Luedke and Harry West and two anonymous reviewers provided insightful and helpful comments on earlier versions of this chapter.

1. With the exception of public figures such as Dr. Ansgar, I have chosen to use pseudonyms for individuals that I mention by name in order to protect their anonymity.
2. Mdunduwaro is a village about ten to fifteen miles away.
3. In the narratives that I heard, the narrators did not refer to this woman by name. They referred to her using generic terms of reference and anonymous

third-person pronouns. I have chosen to use a pseudonym for the sake of clarity and readability.

4. Mgazini is a village on the other side of Mdunduwaro from Peramiho.

5. *UKIMWI* is an acronym that stands for the phrase "*Upungufu wa kinga mwilini*" or "*Ukosefu wa kinga mwilini*" ("reduction in protection/defense in the body")—the Swahili equivalent of Acquired Immune Deficiency Syndrome. In everyday lay Kiswahili, *ukimwi* (which is often lowercased in Swahili-language print media) generally refers both to the HIV virus and to AIDS-related complexes and symptoms, though Tanzanians also refer specifically to the virus (*virusi*) on other occasions. From this point forward, I will use *ukimwi* instead of HIV/AIDS in most cases to signal the importance of Tanzanians' local experiences and understandings of illness.

6. Muhimbili is the national teaching hospital in Dar es Salaam. There is a traditional medicine department attached to Muhimbili.

7. Dr. Ansgar is a German Benedictine monk who serves as medical superintendent at the mission hospital in Peramiho.

8. The term "*bao*" refers to a diagnostic mechanism, often referred to as divination. This mechanism can include a variety of methods involving supernatural means to determine the cause and appropriate treatment for a patient's illness.

9. The rest of the doctors and clinical staff at the hospital were all Tanzanians, and only one other person, a nun who served as a clinical officer, was a member of a religious order. Occasionally expatriate doctors or medical students visited the hospital for relatively short periods of time.

10. The presence, even florescence, of various traditional healing options in the immediate area demonstrates the limitations of this claim. Still, a combination of social and economic power allows the hospital staff and hospital programs to promulgate an almost singular claim to legitimacy and effectiveness in terms of medical treatment. On the relatively few occasions when the hospital chooses to engage traditional healing and traditional healers, the model is almost inevitably one of incorporation rather than mutual cooperation. In contrast to these claims by biomedical representatives, traditional healers give personal accounts that highlight the way both knowledge and patients flow in both directions between biomedicine and traditional healing.

11. Kingoni is the language of Wangoni, who constitute the largest recognized ethnic group in the immediate surrounding area. Members of the older generations tend to speak Kingoni more frequently than others. Adult Wangoni women also speak Kingoni frequently, especially within the household. Kingoni appears to be spoken more widely in less accessible villages.

12. I am grateful to an anonymous reviewer for pointing out the way that this story symbolizes women's generative power.

7 Geographies of Medicine: Interrogating the Boundary between "Traditional" and "Modern" Medicine in Colonial Tanganyika

Stacey Langwick

> A boundary is not that at which something stops but, as the Greeks recognized, the boundary is that from which *something begins its presencing*.
>
> —Martin Heidegger in *Building, Dwelling, Thinking*

Boundaries, Heidegger suggests, are the beginning of all good origin stories. Things do not end at a boundary, they begin there. This chapter explores the history of the boundary between traditional and modern medicine in southeastern Tanganyika.

Under British colonial rule[1] and often specifically through the administration's ties with Christian missions, the practice of biomedicine in Tanganyika was gradually extended beyond urban areas, where it served the health care concerns of colonists and their African laborers, to a broader rural population. During this period, the boundary between biomedicine and so-called traditional medicine emerged as a way to establish certain forms of expertise and authority that were critical to the disciplinary civilizing of colonial modernization. In other words, this boundary served as a solution to particular problems of social order. Such solutions tend to demand solutions to corresponding problems of knowledge.[2] The history of how distinctions between traditional and modern medicine came to be seen as a boundary in Tanganyika is, in a significant sense, the history of how the colonial encounter redefined pluralism.

In the early twentieth century, colonial and mission interventions evoked "traditional medicine" as a category of knowledge that was homogeneous in its opposition to "modern medicine." Later, science—in the form of botanical, chemical, and pharmacological investigations—came to mediate between this dualistic pluralism in a way that further articulated traditional medicine as a discrete and unified category of knowledge enabling targeted intervention. By the mid-1970s, the independent socialist government of Tanzania had started to institutionalize a national traditional medicine that could answer to the same forms of expertise and the same kinds of authority as biomedicine. This chapter examines the expansion of medical practice for the forty years prior to the establishment of postcolonial scientific traditional medicine. By focusing on the expansion of biomedicine in southeastern Tanganyika through the 1930s and 1940s, I illustrate how distinctions among therapies, medicines, and healers came to be fixed as a boundary between traditional medicine and modern medicine in efforts to address problems of social organization.[3]

The work of Leader Stirling, a mission doctor who arrived in British East Africa in 1935 and who later rose to the position of minister of health after independence, offers an illustration of how the boundary between traditional and modern medicine was solidified in Tanzania. In the late 1930s and throughout the 1940s, Stirling established the first broad network of hospitals, clinics, and dispensaries in southeastern Tanganyika. Stirling's accounts offer a unique example of the ways in which rural medical practice came to be ideologically as well as materially invested in the binary between biomedicine and its others. Stirling's forms of description and the structure of his accounts are not neutral. They illustrate attempts to resolve certain challenges to authority in Tanganyika. As such, his representations of the boundary between traditional and modern medicine can be mined for evidence of the ways that the extension of biomedicine to a larger African population participated in redefining healing.[4]

After briefly discussing the narratives that I will draw on in this chapter, I turn more directly to my argument that the representation of the boundary between traditional and modern medicine was an effect of attempts to resolve problems of authority in colonial Tanganyika.[5] First, I examine how Stirling's accounts articulate a landscape in "need" of intervention in order to justify the authority of scientific knowledge. The primacy of the distinction between biomedicine and other ways of treating bodies is possible through the assertion of scientific notions of nature—as that which is to be explained, controlled, and exploited—into descriptions of life and healing in southeastern Tanganyika. Stirling depicts biomedicine (science) as that which has the right to investigate all other forms of therapy (nature). Second, I illustrate how this representation of, and relationship with, nature shapes the space of effective clinical practice. Building projects come to be central to the expansion of biomedicine and, through them, the distinction between traditional and modern medicine is given physicality. Third, I explore boundaries as an effect of the sorting, selecting, gathering, and coordinating of various objects and agents deemed necessary for successful medical practice. Boundaries are inherently unstable. By reclaiming and maintaining this instability in my analysis, I am able to account for the effects of boundary-making. One of the most critical consequences of the boundary between traditional and modern medicine is the separation of healers from botanical medicines, which establishes the ground on which such medicines can be translated into clinical space. The processes that effect the boundary between traditional and modern medicine are the same processes that establish or render present the contours of a scientifically intelligible traditional medicine.

The Doctor's Accounts

I draw primarily from Stirling's published narratives, including two books, *Bush Doctor* (1947) and *Tanzanian Doctor* (1977). I supplement these narratives with comments from a personal interview I conducted with Dr. Stirling in his home after his retirement (2000). My analysis is further shaped by my extended fieldwork in the area where he worked, including conversations with elders who remember Dr. Stirling and his work.

Stirling's first book is a compilation of excerpts from letters he wrote to family and members of the Anglican Church during the first eleven years he spent in Tanganyika. These letters begin in 1935 when, as a newly trained Scottish physician, he embarked for Tanganyika to join the Universities' Mission to Central Africa (UMCA) in the southeastern town of Masasi. He never again returned to the United Kingdom for more than a visit. The letters in this first volume continue through November 1946. After the nation gained independence in 1961, he renounced his British citizenship in order to become a Tanzanian citizen. In 1975, President Julius Nyerere appointed Stirling as the minister of health, a post he held until 1980. During his tenure as minister, his second book, *Tanzanian Doctor,* was published. Much of the content is similar to that of the first. Whole paragraphs, sometimes chapters, are lifted straight from one book to the other, but in this second publication, he continues the story through the mid-1970s. *Tanzanian Doctor,* featuring an introduction by Julius Nyerere, and published by Heinemann in both London and Nairobi, was also an effort to speak in a (slightly) more secular voice to the "outside" world about the steady progress of a recently independent Tanzania. It is a self-conscious marking of a national history through the life of one person who shaped the nation and whose life was itself dramatically shaped through the making of this (at the time) non-aligned socialist African state.

The last few chapters of *Tanzanian Doctor* are about Stirling's participation in the Tanganyikan African National Union (TANU), his work for independence, his position as a member of parliament, and later his role as minister of health. He concludes with reference to his efforts to build a national health care service. Health and healing, hospitals and biomedical objects of therapy, and possible subjectivities and forms of expertise all come to be transformed in the multiple relationships that make up the "encounter" between Europe and Africa during this period.[6] Stirling's narratives and this chapter focus most closely on the moments before Stirling officially became a Tanzanian citizen, when this British colonial mission doctor was in the uneasy position of a colonist refusing to maintain empire.[7] Stirling reworked existing boundaries, not only between European and African, missionary and healer, and colonist and

Tanzanian citizen but also between healers and medicines and families and patients.

Distinctions and Dominations

The history of the emergence of the boundary between traditional and modern medicine in southeastern Tanganyika is part of the larger story of the construction of nature as a scientifically accessible and describable entity. Feminist histories of science have powerfully critiqued the gendered and often violent rhetoric that asserts progress through the domination of nature, which is seen to exist for human benefit and exploitation.[8] Historians of colonialism in Africa have illustrated how various forms of scientific knowledge reshaped the mundane practices and daily patterns of life so they conformed to particularly modernist notions of time and space.[9] Leader Stirling's representation of nature resonates with those critiqued and analyzed by these bodies of work. Stirling's narratives illustrate the ways in which a seemingly inexorable wilderness is asserted as the ground on which colonial distinctions could be made and the efficacy of those distinctions could be evidenced. The landscape in Stirling's accounts is the background for a story of progress. The linear movement of progress can be made visible only against a background of apparent stability. Stirling's way of seeing and describing the landscape of southeastern Tanganyika creates a kind of stability against which he can tell his story of the advancement of the African people through their collaboration with scientific medicine. Other therapies and healers are generally portrayed as an indistinguishable part of this landscape. Only when they are implicated in a particular biomedical struggle do they emerge as defined obstacles, such as poisons or charlatans.

The early chapters in *Tanzanian Doctor* (hereafter *TD*) are full of stories of lions and other wild animals, of long walks, dense forests, and areas deemed "isolated." Missionaries are represented as battling an unruly, unordered, and unmanaged environment. Mission stations offer the hope of taming this (at best) chaotic and (at worst) dangerous wilderness. The existence of these stations, however, is precarious in the face of the "unforgiving forest" where wild animals rule and the forest refuses the effort of more civilized beasts by "swallowing" them (*TD*, 35, 64).

Unlike mission stations, homes and compounds unconnected with the mission are not swallowed by the wilderness; rather, they appear as part of the wilderness, emerging and disappearing in conjunction with it. In Stirling's accounts, the inexorability of the "unforgiving" and "ever-hungry" forest is translated into the mobility of the people he describes. For example, after his first trip to Lulindi, which was to become his base, he writes:

> The soil is often poor, and the ash from the burning was then the only enrichment it ever received. After two years it was exhausted, and the family had to make new fields. If they had a death, or even much sickness, or bad harvests, they would move altogether and build a new village at a distance, to get away from the

influence of local spirits or of there [*sic*] neighbors, who might be thought to
have caused the trouble by charms, spells, and poisons. In this way the shape of
the countryside was constantly changing. Familiar villages quietly disappeared
and were eaten up by the ever-hungry bush, while new clearings and new huts
appeared elsewhere.[10] (*TD*, 14–15)

Common folks are depicted as overwhelmed by other forces. The bush has a
voracious agency and appetite, and the innocent are battered by its growth. In
Stirling's eyes, local farmers fail to stop, contain, or control the wilderness in any
meaningful way. Because the effect of their settlement is rendered insignificant,
the environment (the background to his tale) remains stable even while it is
"constantly changing."

Indeed, those humans with agency in this paragraph are the "neighbors" who
use "charms, spells, and poisons." These neighbors and "local spirits" are in cahoots here with the "ever-hungry" forest. Their ability to move people and
shape the countryside seems to implicate them in nature; they become part of
the wilderness rather than actors against it. From this first introductory trip into
the catchment area of his medical station, Stirling foreshadows the distinction
between missionary-supported biomedicine and other ways of treating misfortunes, discomforts, and bodily concerns. This Other—made homogeneous in its
superstition—will appear as a feature of the environment in which his work
occurs and it will disappear into what Stirling perceives as random, chaotic
nature.

In general, the movement of people from one piece of land to another is
taken as a sign of their vulnerability to broader forces. The inhabitants of this
area are represented as victims of the weather, earth, disease, and beliefs. Yet
some of Stirling's contemporaries left evidence of a more distinct pattern to
people's movement in which land was worked through a three-year cycle of particular crops and then allowed to lie fallow for an extended period of time (some
records say nine years and others twenty).[11] In his passing through, however,
Stirling did not see the patterns of resistance and accommodation that structured people's lives.

The interpretation of the movement of people in this area lies in stark contrast to the representation of Stirling's own extraordinarily mobile lifestyle. The
conscientious doctor was compelled to travel not only to visit hospitals and dispensaries but also to track down reported cases of smallpox when there was an
outbreak and to get medicines and supplies shipped in from Europe. His account is filled with amazing stories of fixing cars and ambulances, rescuing
them from muddy bogs and overflowing rivers, bicycling long distances, and
trekking tirelessly. Describing his routine in 1936, he writes:

I usually stay a week or ten days at one station, and then move on, doing anything
up to twenty-seven miles a day on foot, or more with the help of a bike. A day's
walk usually brings one to the next station with a dispensary or hospital, but sometimes it may take two or three days from one to another. (*Bush Doctor*, hereafter
BD, 45)

The doctor, with the untiring vigilance expected only of a savior, is pitted against the elements. The bad roads, the rainy season and resulting raging rivers, the malarial mosquitoes, the heat and fog and thickets and other whims of nature are things he consistently conquers. His domination is enacted not only through the achievement of his specific goals (to get to a sick patient, to move medicines to a remote clinic, etc.) but also through his writing about them as personal interest stories in an otherwise dry bureaucratic tale of the "inevitable" expansion of biomedicine.

Of course, the position from which Stirling was seeing shaped not only how he described the environment but also how he described the disposition of people living there. For instance, on the Makonde Plateau, another part of Stirling's district, where he later established a substantial hospital and several smaller dispensaries, he perceived wildness and wilderness as explicitly working against (his) clarity and sight. He represents the "density" of the bush as obscuring and misleading. He describes the bush of the "plateau country" as

> so dense that only a wild pig could penetrate it, and growing to the height of ten feet or more it effectively shut out all view of the surrounding country from the slot-like paths and roads. The paths tended to become tunnels. One could drive for miles through this bush without sight of a house, thus having the quite false impression that the country was uninhabited. Actually the bush was honeycombed with paths leading to hamlets in small clearings, and was one of the most densely populated areas in Tanganyika. (*TD*, 18)

Stirling does not ask whose sight is obscured, who is given "false impressions," or from what perspective the view is "shut out." For him, the "endless expanse of secondary bush" does not (as it may very well have for many people living in the area) allow one to know when visitors are coming before they officially arrive to announce themselves. His bush does not frame pathways or establish the safety of homesteads. Since the people in this area had earlier been fleeing from Ngoni raiders to the West, they would likely have seen the height of the plateau and the density of the bush as a benefit to their resistance and survival.[12] We can well imagine that their depiction of what the bush obscured and revealed would have been quite different. Ways of seeing are not natural; the way the natural is seen is historical and political.

While Stirling's strongly modernist and practical narrative does not often allow itself abstract reflection, in a 1941 letter to distant family, Stirling does link the domination of nature to distinctions in space and time. He writes that "life remains much as usual—the endless struggle with the devil and the forces of nature, in a land where space is unlimited and time unconsidered—but pleasant enough on the surface" (*BD*, 89–90). For those who can see beyond the surface of everyday life with the X-ray vision of religion and modernity, he implies, all is not pleasant underneath. Rather, festering there is an interminable hell where time is unconsidered because nothing ever changes,[13] where space is limitless because there is no beyond, and where all is ruled by the devil. Here is our stable background—a wilderness of such unlimited, unconsidered hunger that it has devoured all the markings of time and space. "Life as usual" is dangerously fluid, an excess that cannot be marked because there is no point of overflowing. His job, and that of his colleagues, is to limit space and to consider time. Health—as it existed for Stirling, his biomedical contemporaries, and his modern, mostly European audience—demanded the creation of boundaries.

Initiating Boundaries

The struggle to negotiate these temporal and spatial boundaries in the complicated array of interests, desires, objects, and actors concerned with bodies and well-being in southeastern Tanganyika is illustrated particularly clearly in the issues surrounding boys' circumcisions. Initiation ceremonies, he writes:

> occurred about every third year, and involved the segregation of all the uninitiated boys and girls into secret camps. The boys were kept in the forest. . . . The circumcisions were carried out in completely primitive and barbaric fashion, the boys lying in the dust surrounded by a howling, yelling mob, while fierce drumming drowned their cries. Naturally there was always much trouble afterwards, from septic wounds, haemorrhage, and other complications. (*TD*, 47)

"Howling boys," "a yelling mob," and "fierce drumming" in a forest of "secrets," "dirt," and "confusion." It was impossible to see, and "utterly impossible" to administer, "useful treatment." "Naturally there was . . . trouble," and the trouble was marked with naturalized scientific terms: septic wounds and hemorrhage. The good doctor, however, finds that all too easily his efforts can slip into feeding (rather than fighting) the hunger of this chaotic wilderness. He recounts:

> [T]he idea had got about that it was a good thing to ask the doctor and his assistants to come along and apply some European dressings to the wounds. I consequently attended a number of these circumcisions, but found the conditions utterly impossible for applying any useful treatment, owing to the indescribable dirt and confusion that prevailed. The problem was made more difficult by the fact that the Mission had given its blessing to these ceremonies, in an expurgated form, and the mission hospital was expected to give full support. This encouragement also increased the popularity of these rites, at a time when in other areas they were rapidly dying out. (*TD*, 47–48)

Over the first six years of his medical work, Stirling and his assistants "examined and treated 1,000 boys in these initiation camps" and "tried every means . . . to bring order out of chaos and to establish some sort of antiseptic regime." During this time, he and his medical staff offered, and sometimes were granted permission, to conduct the circumcisions themselves in the camps, thereby controlling at least the most immediate instruments in the act of cutting. "But," he concludes, "the conditions were utterly impossible, and in the end I could only urge that all boys should be brought to hospital for circumcision" (*TD*, 48). This image of impossible chaos renders invisible the distinctions that were critical to these initiations. Stirling does not recognize boundaries that shape these initiation camps, such as those between forest and village, men and women, the spiritual and the mundane. Through his depiction of an undifferentiated morass, he confirms the stability of the wilderness. His ineffectiveness comes to imply that all effective action requires that the wilderness itself must first be controlled.

In contrast, those organizing the initiations at this time appear to have taken a different position than Stirling. They assumed that the greater number of threatening entities, whether ancestors or bacteria, being engaged and controlled (within the boundaries of the camp), the better. Initiation leaders were less concerned with distinctions between "modern" and "traditional" medicine; they invited hospital doctors to bring their "antiseptic regime" and all the actors and agents that this involved into the camps. Stirling, however, could find no way to negotiate the plurality of this relationship. He could not manipulate threatening bacteria in the spaces of ancestors and spirits. Apparently, what these ancestors required for engagement worked against what Stirling's bacteria required for engagement. "In the end," Stirling insists that biomedical practices must be an alternative to these "traditional practices." He resists participation in these ceremonies.

The move to the hospital privileged the physical boundary between biomedicine and the outside environment, in this case the chaos of the forest initiation. Working together in the forest would have necessitated the enactment of more complex and subtle connections between biomedical and nonbiomedical practitioners. Arguing that the mission should remove itself from the forest was a process of arguing against the importance of these connections. One can imagine a different response from that of Stirling. Indeed, the UMCA bishop and other church leaders were at this time promoting collaboration and lobbying against Stirling's kind of binarism. The boundary then emerges as an effect of resisting connection.

This resistance was not simply the result of stubbornness. The boundaries of the clinic were critical to the agency of Stirling and his colleagues—not just the boundaries that were constituted through the fences and walls of the hospital but also all the forms of order and visible representations of objects that became possible and comprehensible only behind those fences and walls. The infrastructure of the hospital and the spatial-conceptual distinctions it involved were critical to the healing power of biomedical practitioners.

Building, Healing, Thinking

While the struggle over boys' bodies and health during initiations illustrates the importance of space to effective healing practice, such descriptions of engaged conflict with "traditional" practitioners are rare in Stirling's accounts. In his heroic tales of the early expansion of biomedicine through an area of health disasters, Stirling describes little direct antagonism or competition between himself and his staff and those who advocate other therapeutic practices. When the plants, minerals, dances, consultations, and other elements used to care for disordered, dysfunctional, or uncomfortable bodies in southern Tanganyika do surface in Stirling's narratives, they are described more often as obstacles in a nature that is perceived as unruly and problematic than as an alternative way of healing. This lack of conflict is critical to the administrative and clinical effort of advocates of biomedicine in the first two-thirds of the twentieth century to refigure healing in a way that centralized that practice (first definitionally and then structurally).

In fact, nonbiomedical ways of healing hardly seem to be present to Stirling. He constructs his narratives to build a sense of significant unmet need. For example, he writes:

> Besides building up the two main hospitals [in the late 1930s], I was opening up more dispensaries in strategic places. With medical aide so scarce these dispensaries filled a great need. . . . One of these new dispensaries was at Mkunya, on the Makonde plateau, so placed that it was able to take over work from overpressed Newala and Mahuta, and also save sick people many weary miles traveling. (*TD*, 58)

One might argue convincingly that such a tone is merely practical since the text is only slightly modified from that which was originally intended for the church society and family and friends back home who might support the expansion of facilities. Statistics on numbers of patients and descriptions of large crowds of people waiting to be treated are also frequent parts of the storyline. I suggest, however, that the desire or intention to appeal to potential financial contributors is only part of the effect of this representation of scarcity and need. Stirling's narrative strategy mimics that of earlier explorers; the difference is that now *healing* is the virgin territory. There is in this narrative little sense of collaboration, coordination, or even competition with other forms of healing because there is little sense that other (effective) therapies are available. The empty therapeutic landscape—a wilderness of sick and suffering—awaited European intervention.

Building becomes one of the key interventions, the answer to wilderness of all kinds: natural, religious, and human. Leader Stirling's accounts are dominated by descriptions of the interventions he directed to structurally extend biomedicine throughout southeastern Tanganyika. His letters and stories are filled with the buildings he hopes to build or the buildings he is designing, improving, supervising, constructing, or having dedicated. Although medical boundaries were definitely ideological, they were not merely metaphorical. They had the hard edges of brick walls, aluminum roofing, concrete floors, and fencing.

Building a network of hospitals and dispensaries required a domestication of the landscape and the construction of ever-more permanent and less "earthy" structures. Nature and the disorder of the African environment are constantly creeping in on medical work, even outside the initiation camps. Stirling describes lumps of dirt and grass falling into a patient's open wound as she was being operated on (*TD*, 38). In 1938, after reflecting on the completion of the year's extensive building work, Stirling looks forward, suggesting his plans for the next year. He worries: "So there is still plenty to do, and even more at Newala as there the operating theatre is only a mud house and that is being eaten by white ants" (*BD*, 64). Stirling quickly assures his English audience that when the operating theater in Lulindi suddenly fell down because it was "only a bamboo building . . . it was cleared away, and now we are building a proper operation-block" (*BD*, 48). This plot is common in Stirling's vignettes; over and over again, the protagonist, the proper building, answers the antagonist, the wilderness.

What is this proper building? In the 1936 rebuilding of the Lulindi operating theater, it was characterized by

> walls of sun-dried mud bricks, with a floor of stone and the usual grass roof. Novel features include a roof of sugarcane board (it will be the only ceiling in the district!), a proper ventilation though air filters, glass windows, and permanent lighting from two paraffin-vapour lamps, inverted type, each of 400 candle power. There is to be a sterilizing room at one end and two ante-rooms at the other, one for preparation of the patient, anaesthetic, etc. and one for the recovery of the same. (*BD*, 48)

Two aspects of the proper building come to define its "properness": its construction materials and its division of space by time or process.

"Properness" is partly constituted through the ability of various building materials to resist "nature," which for Stirling is tied to the amount of processing involved in their transformation from "raw" products. In the description of the Lulindi operating theater above, sun-dried bricks are championed in an implicit comparison with the more common mud and wattle. Later, Stirling announces the coming of even-more-proper fired bricks. In addition, the floor is of cut stone rather than dirt. Air is regulated and filtered. The coming of night does not mean darkness. Glass windows let in the sunshine but not dirt and insects. Through these processes of separating, filtering, blocking, and eliminating, the wilderness is constructed as the outside and as that which is full of contagions and threats. Later, Stirling reflects on the thatched roof—grass tied to bamboo poles with strong forest materials—as the Achilles' heel of the proper building in these initial incarnations. Thatch "gets blown about by whirlwinds, it leaks, it harbours rats, snakes, and white ants, and always there is the danger of fire; with thatch this means the end of the house and everything in it" (*TD*, 40). It was not effective in repelling the wilderness, whether it came as rain, wind, or animal. Stirling's "proper building" evolves over time, responding to the various threats that turn the plot for our history. Later, it acquires roofing tiles.

The second characteristic of our protagonist the "proper building," which is essential to shaping the way it evolved through time, is its effectiveness in establishing the boundaries that define the subjects and objects of medical practices. The physical borders and boundaries that delineate hospital space are not just repressive bulwarks against such things as wilderness; they are also creative. The protagonist compels the staff to enter through the sterilizing room and the patients to enter through a special prep room. The proper building guides the movement of other actors. In its resistance to the "ever-hungry wilderness," it forms spaces that assist in shaping patients' bodies as objects of biomedical practice and positioning doctors and nurses as subjects acting on these bodies. The preparation of patients, the act of surgery, and the period of recovery came to be distinguishable not only through activities and states (that might be just as easily seen as blending seamlessly into one another) but also through the space the patient inhabited. Proper buildings first emerge in these narratives in the form of "operating blocks," a group of rooms designed for the preparation for and practice of surgery. The surgical procedures that transform individual bodies into appropriate objects of therapeutic practice include not only stripping them of contagions through preparation but also stripping them, in significant ways, of their "culture" (including beliefs, suspicions, and preferred alternatives) through anaesthetization. Although we will see below that the body being operated on is far from universal, the operating theater emerges again and again as a critical site for the negotiated emergence of biomedical objects of practice and intervention. In these negotiations, proper buildings have a form of agency.[14]

The frustration Stirling felt in the initiation camps was not present in the clinical buildings he constructed, at least partly because the proper building worked to isolate the subjects and objects critical to biomedical practice. These subjects and objects, which included "the patient" and health care practitioners such as "the nurse," emerge in part through their distinction from "family." Initially, Stirling finds that families insist on being in the operating room with their relative undergoing a surgical procedure in order to "make sure that bits of the patient were not taken away to be made into 'medicine' for use in witchcraft" (*TD*, 41). Over time he deals with this complication through architectural design. Just as he had constructed buildings with corrugated iron roofing or tiles to keep the thatch from falling down at inopportune times, and just as he organized the making of bricks to improve on flimsy bamboo structures, he also slowly builds the family out of the operating room. He writes that he "was able to reduce family representation to two and then to one, who had to be properly garbed in cap and mask and sit quietly in a corner." Later, he "inserted a special window, so that the relatives could sit in an ante-room and watch all that went on in the theatre" (*TD*, 41). Boundaries become ever-more solid, from the cloth of caps and masks to the materials of walls and windows. Stirling tells his readers that by the 1970s, few family members "trouble[d]" to watch their relatives under the knife anymore. In this example, the proper building, in collaboration with so many other agencies, is deemed to have done its job.

Stirling defines biomedical patients not only through the architecture of the operating theater but also through the architecture of the ward. In 1944, when Stirling adds the first hospital wards in the area to the Lulindi hospital, he is anxious about the response to the greater definition of the "patient" and the "nurse" this new version of the proper building facilitated. He writes:

> To have patients nursed in actual wards and not in small houses, is an entirely new development here, and therefore it will be experimental. Hitherto all patients have been fed and cared for by their own relations, with consequently a lot of mess and

often to the detriment of such treatment and nursing as we try to give, but the system has its advantages in that we have been able to deal with a large number of patients with a small staff, and without having to worry about feeding them. I have no idea therefore of suddenly changing the system for the whole hospital, but by providing for a maximum of twenty patients in the new wards we can see how it will work, and then if successful, we can build more wings to the hospital and gradually extend until all in-patients are being *properly* nursed and fed. (emphasis mine, *BD*, 121)

In caring for their relatives, family members were literally crossing the boundary from town, village, and forest into the hospital. This crossing brought with it all kinds of other possibilities for crossings, not the least of which for Stirling was the carrying of germs, ticks, fleas and the like onto the hospital grounds. As families were cooking, bathing, and caring for their sick relatives, there were many possible points where the standards of hygiene, patient compliance with taking medicine, or the regularity with which dressings were changed could be less rigorous than he would have desired. Families also brought other ideas. Their confidences as well as fears had to be negotiated with those of the patient. Traditional medicines could easily travel with family members onto the hospital grounds and (unofficially) into the medical treatment regime of the patient. Families were, in short, "a lot of mess" and a "detriment" to nursing care. Many (f)actors had to come together to negotiate the separation of a patient from his family. One of the first, and the one foregrounded here by Stirling, is the rallying of a new version of the proper building. The walls and screens of these first wards not only shape a particular kind of patient but also structure proper nursing and proper feeding. Boundaries allow for the distinction between improper family care and improper feeding with the care and feeding by trained hospital staff. The proper building does not work by itself but as part of a broader collective of actors. The actors who designed, constructed, and worked in the operating blocks and hospital wards in southeastern Tanganyika both shaped those buildings and were shaped by them. In Stirling's accounts, the agency of the proper building is illustrated most clearly as it shapes the biomedical subject-object known as the patient.

Making the claim that there was a "great need" for European medicines and expertise was a critical narrative move in the expansion of biomedicine in Tanganyika—a move that was made both to mark progress and to justify its altruistic civilizing mission. In such claims, the therapeutic landscape was represented as bare and no local medicines seemed to threaten the justification for medical colonialism. Other medicines and therapies, of course, not only existed but were impossible to completely ignore. In other narratives by colonial doctors, healers are important (even if understated) interlocutors in the establishment of biomedical clinics and dispensaries.[15] Although Stirling gives no space to individual healers, as Iliffe has suggested, no doctor or biomedical institution could ignore the fact that patients came with expectations of what medicine was and what it meant to be treated, with fears of particular threats, with convictions about nameable agents, and (sometimes) with their bodies full of herbal medicines.[16] Stirling lamented the fact that many people arrived at the hospital with very complicated case histories because they had been treated by traditional healers (*TD*, 44). He also claimed that some patients arrived suffering more from the effects of a poison given to them by a "medicine-man" than from the effects of any illness (*TD*, 44–45). Herbal medicines and poisons and witchcraft are almost interchangeable in his account. They all participate in creating a vague sense that there are features of African life that must be overcome, managed, or built out of medicine in Tanganyika. The target of such efforts, however, is not particular therapies or treatments but rather the family.

Transgression or Mediation?

Not all challenges to biomedicine could be resolved through a strengthening of boundaries. Because patients themselves could not be built out of hospital medicine, creative accommodations to some of the challenges they posed were also necessary. Families and buildings surface again. In contrast, they appear in this section not as sites for the production of boundaries between biomedicine and "the wilderness out there" but rather as sites of complicated negotiations and translations between biological and nonbiological threats to life and livelihood. Priests sprinkled Christian "medicine" on new hospital wards to protect them from evil spirits and witchcraft, while families, with or without their caps and masks, were sometimes allies rather than obstacles. The walls of the hospital and the boundaries between the binaries of modernist thought are also sites of interaction, translation, and exchange.

Through structures of consent and the possible repercussions of blame, the family remained constitutive of the patient even when relatives were outside their viewing stations in the operating theater. In a discussion of the difficulties of surgery in southeastern Tanganyika, Stirling writes:

> Besides the patient's natural fear of an operation there was the complication that any injury to an individual was in African eyes an injury to the family, and so before an operation could be done not only was the consent of the patient essential but also that of all his relatives. Even if the patient were willing, the obstinate refusal of some old man, or even more often some old woman, would often make it impossible to operate, and one had to watch the patient dying slowly of a condition that could easily have been relieved. (*TD*, 40–41)

The structures of family, ideas about personhood, different objects of therapy, and lines of authority that made up life outside the hospital grounds were not clearly separated from biomedicine even after trust in the hospital staff increased and fear that they were using body parts for harmful purposes decreased. The "obstinate refusals" of old men and woman to allow relatives to undergo operations were stubborn reminders of the defining presence of nonbiomedical relationships of person and body that were inseparable from the patient.

Mission medicine and local constructions of family and person were not neatly opposed, however. Stirling not only describes how relatives and old chiefs at times refused to allow a willing patient to undergo treatment, he also describes how, at other times, they insisted on treatment for an unwilling patient. Stirling notes blithely that "[o]ccasionally this collective responsibility had its uses." Then he gives an example of "a woman [who] refused an urgent operation, but her family decided she should have it, and ignoring her screams of protest they carried her bodily into the theatre and held her body down until she was anaesthetized" (*TD*, 41). The family bursts into the operating block, and suddenly in the service of surgery they become welcome allies.

Others who suddenly appeared at the operating table were less welcome. Through the treatment of another female patient, Stirling suddenly found himself in cahoots with what he saw as unsavory charlatans.

> Another woman came from further away, beyond the Ruvuma[,] with a hard mass that felt like a fibroid uterus. I operated, but when I tried to deliver the uterus in the ordinary way, it jumped right out on the table. It was no uterus at all, but a very large solid fibroma of one ovary. This was very easy to remove, and I took it along later to show the patient. I thought she would be pleased, but she didn't even smile. She gave the tumour a very sour look, and said with real hatred in her voice, "Now I'm going to find out who put that thing in my belly." She disappeared soon after without paying her modest bill (operations were only 1s. each in those days) and probably spent large sums to pin the tumour, by divination, on some wretched neighbor. The tumour may well have caused endless suspicion and maltreatment of quite innocent people, and it might have been better if I had never removed it. (*TD*, 41–42)

Like the family above, this tumor seems to burst into the operating theater, but this surprise guest was not an ally, for it brought with it the trace of a diviner.

Nonbiomedical experts, medicines, and interpretations occasionally seem to burst through the boundaries of modern medicine. Stirling describes these moments that acknowledge other ways of treating bodies and their various states through strangely truncated stories, which he does not link to the narrative that comes before or after. Stirling's vignettes of intruding others are told as short bursts in themselves. Frequently, they are offered up with a note of mirth. Their oddly partial telling is critical both to the sense that there is a boundary around modern medicine and that it is holding back certain things. The separation of biomedicine from all that is outside the hospital grounds creates both a specifically situated lack and its corollary, a teaming wilderness. The sudden appearance of objects that resist refiguring and narrative turns that go nowhere heighten the sense that the out-there is bursting through to the in-here. These accounts convey a sense of boundary through descriptions of transgression. Paradoxically then, Stirling articulates the fixity of the distinction between traditional and modern medicine through his representation of porous boundaries—that is, those that are vulnerable to transgression.

Such porousness accounts for difference and anomaly. It explains away times of inconsistency. Porousness, in Stirling's memoirs, serves as deviance did for his more academic contemporaries. In the 1930s, only a couple of years before Stirling first put his foot on Tanganyikan soil, English translations of Durkheim's work were being published and the influence of Talcott Parsons was beginning to shape a redefinition of (particularly American) sociology. In structural functionalist analyses, public repercussions for those who crossed normative boundaries functioned as a social reminder or reinforcement of those boundaries. The conventions through which Stirling represents alternative ways of healing offers them up to the reader as similar mechanisms of regulatory control.

Those who seek the assistance of healers before coming to the hospital are likely to suffer for their transgression, such as the man with only one foot who crawled up to the dispensary. After a puff-adder bite, this man had developed gangrene. As he was pulling himself along the fifteen miles or so to the dispensary his foot dropped off in the road. In telling the story of this patient, Stirling claims that

> these cases respond well to simple surgical principles (elevation of the leg with absolute rest, incision and hypertonic compresses, antibiotics, vasodilators and morphia) and with this regime I had never seen gangrene develop. It develops readily enough, however, in those who walk about looking for anti-snake medicine. There are many local remedies for snakebite, their chief aim being to make the victim vomit. From the pathology of snakebite it is highly improbable that any of them has any useful effect, the high recovery rate being due to the non-poisonous character of most local snakes. (*TD*, 93)

This poor man paid with his foot for not knowing or not believing that biomedical treatment could cure him. Stirling not only blames his boundary-crossing—"walk(ing) about looking for anti-snake medicine"—for his permanent disfigurement, he also claims that it is "improbable" that any such crossing would be efficacious. This is not as much an illustration for rural Tanzanians who were vulnerable to puff-adder bites as a reinforcement of the boundary between biomedicine and other forms of treating threats and discomforts for his mostly European audience.

Bruno Latour's studies of the production of scientific knowledge give us a particularly effective way to approach these all-too-brief appearances of other treatment regimes. Latour has argued that processes of purification and mediation are critical moves for those who are (never quite) modern. The purification of an in-here from an out-there, of the observer from the observed, of self from other, of interpretation or explanation from the "real world" is in some sense the project of modernity. Equally central to the moderns, however, is the process of negotiating or mediating between these distinct (or purified) entities. That is, processes that effect the fixity of boundary (purification) are only one aspect of the processes that produce new categories of knowledge and the subjects and objects that inhabit them. Stirling may not be interested in seeing how surgery gives rise to new ways of identifying the work of *wachawi* (sorcerers); however, he is willing and eager to have hospital buildings protected from evil spirits.

Stirling's narrative privileges some forms of mediation. Following Latour, we might examine when and how processes of purification or processes of medication are used.

In 1936, Stirling wrote that the new Masasi out-patient building was "blessed and dedicated to the glory of God and the honour of All Saints . . . because so many of the patients (heathen) live in much constant fear of evil spirits and attribute all their illnesses thereto" (*BD*, 40). Almost three years later, when the bishop blessed a new building in Lulindi, Stirling described the ceremony as follows:

> We all went in procession to the hospital and stood in front of it while the Bishop went all round the building, both outside and inside sprinkling holy water. Then, standing in the doorway, he said the traditional prayers, exorcising any evil spirits, and praying for God's blessing on the building and all the work to be done there, finally placing it under the special protection of St. Michael the Archangel. Some of you might think that such a ceremony is old fashioned and quite unnecessary, but in this land at least it has a very real significance. The people here go in constant fear of evil spirits and witches, and even when they become Christians it is one of the hardest things for them to overcome and to realize that the Holy Spirit is stronger than all. So to know that the house has been solemnly blessed in the name of Almighty God, and that therefore no evil spirit can enter in, is to give a great increase of confidence, and this is especially important in a hospital. Most illness is ascribed to evil spirits or witches, and the removal of this fear is of first importance. (*BD*, 73)

Stirling talks of evil spirits and witches not as actors but as fears, as "one of the hardest things for them to overcome." Furthermore, the ceremony seems, in his view, to have given "a great increase of confidence" rather than prevented such dangerous threats from entering into the building. Such dedications were specific attempts to mediate between the actors who were important to patients (such as *wachawi* and their threatening medicines, ancestors, and numerous other "spirits" who could inflect harm) and the objects of therapy that were important to biomedical doctors (such as parasites, worms, and tumors).

The play between purification and mediation is critical. Nonscientific entities were engaged by the church and the clinic only in an effort to bring medicine to more people and to establish more places to combat scientific threats. If mediation did not appear to address these goals, then it was to be avoided, as Stirling insisted in 1939.

> The Newala hospital was opened by the District Officer on the Feast of the Epiphany after being blessed by the priest-in-charge. There was a large crowd of people, including the Indian shopkeepers who are pretty numerous at Newala and who contributed generously to the building, enabling us to have a concrete floor which would otherwise have been impossible. The D.O. made a good speech and then flung open the doors and was escorted in. Someone suggested that he should publicly drink the first dose of medicine[,] preferably castor oil. And I believe that he would meekly have done so, but I put my foot down firmly! (*BD*, 74)

Perhaps such public medicine-taking resonated with witchcraft eradication movements a little too strongly. These movements required all people in a village or area to take certain medicines designed to ensure that communities were protected against witchcraft. In this process, individuals were given medicines that would have killed them if they were to commit acts of witchcraft. Witchcraft eradication movements emerged in southern Tanganyika after the German colonial administration crushed the Maji Maji Rebellion in 1907, and waves of witchcraft eradication still existed in the 1930s.[17] I have found evidence of such public efforts to address the fears of and dangers of witches in southeastern Tanzania up to 1995. In addition, I have often seen a *mganga* or healer take her own medicines, particularly protective medicines, in order to prove her belief in their potency and/or their gentleness (*baridi*). Whatever historical and contemporary echoes helped to generate this call to take medicine, it is interesting that Stirling chose to put his "foot firmly down" at this point. For him, a relevant conceptual boundary existed here. If the colonial district administrator had drunk castor oil as part of the ceremony to open the new hospital, it would not have been a move to substitute the Holy Spirit for other medicines, and it would not have been an opportunity to see the Holy Spirit as stronger than other agents and actors in the area. Rather, this drinking of castor oil would have implicated the hospital, and the church to the extent that folks connected the two, in a relationship with healers. It seems that the importance of this conceptual boundary may not have been as important to the district commissioner.

Hospital walls are the sites of negotiations between evil spirits and poisonous snakebites and between angry ancestors or common parasites. When boundaries are not the markers of ahistorical or natural differences but rather the effect of a long series of accommodations and resistances, the way(s) that these negotiations are to be resolved is (are) not always predictable. In this sense, boundaries might be said to be inherently unstable even if they are heavy under the weight of history. Reading boundaries as the effect of combined practices of purification and mediation reclaim (at least some of) the agency behind the making of these distinctions. It allows us to see the Heideggerian "something" that this boundary-making "presenced."

Contours of Traditional Medicine

A great deal of time, energy, and materials went into purifying the space of biomedicine from all that was not deemed scientific or modern. Nevertheless, nonbiomedical objects of treatment (e.g., bodily masses produced by *uchawi*, or witchcraft) and substances of therapies (e.g., herbal medicines taken before coming to the hospital or brought by relatives) entered the clinic. While responses to such encounters varied, some moves to purify and mediate objects of healing, substances of treatment, experts, and institutional relationships generated references to "traditional medicine." Such mediations actively circumscribed the ways in which botanical, mineral, and animal products were acknowledged in the clinic. This section turns specifically to those moves that identified traditional medicine and negotiated new boundaries between healers and therapies.

In a chapter called "The Problems of Insanity and Paralysis," Stirling describes a patient who was taken "to a local herbalist, who confined her in conditions of the utmost squalor and dosed her with the most revolting concoctions containing peoples' spittle and other disgusting ingredients. Naturally she got no better" (*TD*, 111–112). For most colonial doctors, the "local herbalist" was an obstacle, not a colleague. Dr. Stirling was perhaps more generous than most when he confessed that he had an easier time convincing people on the Makonde Plateau to undergo operations that he recommended because "they used to do their own surgery after a fashion." However, his skepticism and even condescension regarding this "surgery" was clear as he continued by saying: "They used to chop each other about. Not very skillfully, but they had the best of intentions" (interview 2000). The by now well-critiqued tone of condescension by a colonist is not the interesting point here. Rather, what enables Stirling's narrative position is the similarity he draws between his work and the work of healers. Both are, in this case, "surgery." By using the category of surgery to rhetorically connect various practices of cutting through the skin, Stirling distinguishes individual healers from abstract practices. This separation renders him as a surgeon fit to judge the therapies of other practitioners as good or bad, desirable or undesirable, efficacious or inefficacious.

Stirling depicted "so-called healers" as "entirely unscientific" and "commercial." He was critical of their techniques and evaluated them as "painful" and often "ineffective." He was wary of their medicines, claiming that they were untested at best and poisonous at worst. Therefore, even though Stirling admitted that "the average patient went to two or three so-called healers first," this was a burden ("we used to get neglected and complicated cases"), not an opportunity for coordination. Of course, hospital doctors typically saw patients for whom nonbiomedical treatments did not "work," because people who went from the healer's home to the hospital were generally motivated by the feeling that their condition had continued to be untenable even after the healer's treatment. Yet he claimed that all healers' diagnoses and treatment were "guesswork." It was possible that a person's complaint might be addressed by an appropriate herbal medicine, but in Stirling's view, those rare occasions happened by coincidence or good luck, not because healers understood the natural arrangements and relations of a scientific world. Therapeutic improvement was, in such cases, an accident. Stirling opposed healers and their intentions to doctors and the modern scientific biomedicine they practice.

In Stirling's writing, the untrustworthy problematic healer was juxtaposed with the possibility of scientifically intelligible and useful herbal medicines. Botanicals mediated the boundary between traditional and modern therapies. Although he expressed a sense that some roots, herbs, or minerals might have medicinal properties, only one extended passage in Stirling's writing discussed a particular nonbiomedical organic medicine. In this paragraph, some of the binaries discussed above were at play, as were gestures toward the processes of purification that allowed them to be mobilized. In addition, Stirling illustrated ways in which things, such as plant matter, were transformed as they were strategically moved across the divisions these binaries created. To narratively establish these already-made-pure forms, he prefaced his account with dire warnings against healers who were not men of science. Only then did he concede that "there is no doubt that some of these medicines are valuable" and claim that he was "able to test and approve at least one." At that point, he tells the following story:

> A child was brought with a large burn on one thigh, and I saw that the burn had been coated with a sticky substance. This was not unusual, as most burns had received some first-aid application, often lamp oil or honey. In this case, however, the appearance was quite impressive, so instead of cleaning off the medicine I simply applied some dry gauze and bandaged it. After ten days I gently peeled off the gauze, and saw a perfectly clean, healed, area of skin. (*TD*, 45)

Stirling's "test," however, did not rely on observation only. Presumably, people in Africa have long assessed therapies by checking the improvement of wounds after the application of a medicine. Stirling's test, then, also required the conjecture that the treatment was translated into a chemical ingredient. He says:

> On enquiring I found that this application was latex from the bark of a tree called *mtomoni*. It obviously contained plenty of tannic acid, and was also a strong adhesive. These two constituents made a most effective coagulation-dressing (this was long before tannic acid had come into disrepute) and I subsequently recommended *mtomoni* for burns in my first-aid instructions to the Scouts. (*TD*, 45–46)

Because the bark of the *mtomoni* tree contains tannic acid and is an adhesive, it becomes comprehensible to a man of science. In this translation, it moved across the set of binaries: from magic to science, from poison or irritant to medicine, from a resource of African healers to a resource of European doctors, from obstacle to solution. Older local lineages of healing and their experts still have no place in Stirling's account. Unruly African herbals, however, may cross over categorical boundaries through the process of being measured, analyzed, and "tested"; that is, in a sense, domesticated. Its value, however, remains a "primitive" solution to the problems of the medicinal mission. Stirling considered this medicine an innovative local addition to the survival first aid taught to Boy Scouts.

Even as he allowed tannic acid to mediate between traditional and modern medicine, Stirling moved to purify these categories of medicine again. Without any ado (even a paragraph break), he informed his readers: "These herbal medicines and their associated charms are used for many purposes beside illness, in fact for almost any of life's problems whether domestic, social, commercial, or anything else" (*TD*, 46). One particular organic material applied to burns moves swiftly to produce an undifferentiated category of the Other.

Then, in a narrative turn that leaves the impression that these others are neither generally comprehensible to science and biomedicine nor particularly threatening, Stirling offered the following vignette:

> A local chief had a grudge against an elderly deacon, so he secreted a packet of medicine in the roof of the deacon's house. Before long a whirlwind completely removed the thatch, but the deacon felt his enemy had been worsted, as the medicine in the roof was now exposed to public view and the chief was thus put to public shame. In other words, loss of face is worse than loss of thatch. (*TD*, 46)

In an attempt to bring harm to this elderly deacon, the local chief had tucked *uchawi*, medicines that call on agents of mischief and death, under his eaves. Still today, whirlwinds are often thought to be a manifestation of harmful actors. Therefore, many might have seen the medicine as working. However, in Stirling's narrative, the churchman triumphs over the local chief-cum-medicine man because his medicines were detected. It is likely that others read this incident with more ambivalence. This revelation may have inspired fear in the chief's subjects in addition to the disgust or anger that might have led to public shaming. By contrasting this story of using medicine to bring harm to another with his account of the tannic acid, Stirling establishes science as the moral arbiter, deciding to link traditional medicine either to witchcraft or to biomedicine. In this way, his representational conventions cover up any ambivalence among unscientific others. Here, echoing our earlier discussion of the nature Stirling described, we readers are given a vignette of victory over the local environment—human and otherwise.

The binary distinctions in Stirling's narratives were fixed into the landscape through his work. Walls, clinical practitioners, and hospital policies excluded healers, ancestors, spirits, harmful intentions and jealousies, bewitched snakes, and other scientifically unintelligible actors from the clinical space. Stirling represented the effect of these exclusions, and of carefully mediated transgressions, as a boundary.

Boundary is not just a metaphor through which difference can be described; the declaring and enforcing of a boundary also resolves problems of authority and social order through the articulation of particular differences. The politics of boundaries lie within the history of their emergence and their maintenance.

The salience of the distinction between biomedicine and all other ways of addressing discomforts, misfortunes, and disabilities is a product of the global spread and institutional privileging of biomedicine. Diverse therapies were lumped together and made homogeneous through their opposition to modern medicine. In 1976, when Leader Stirling was minister of health, the research Institute of Traditional Medicine was established at Muhimbili, the primary government hospital in Tanzania. Since its inception, this institute has been staffed with ethnopharmacologists, chemists, botanists, and (more recently) a social scientist rather than healers. In 1996, an Office of Tanzanian Traditional Medicine was established within the Ministry of Health, and biomedically trained personnel have run that as well. Healers in Tanzania today are confronted by a contemporary category of traditional medicine. They are asked to register themselves with the government and to swear that they are not involved in matters of witchcraft. As some of the chapters in this volume illustrate, non-biomedical healers often find power in reformulating or crossing these very boundaries. The historical comparisons, alignments, connections, and separations that effect the boundary between traditional and modern medicine continue to redefine what healing is in Tanzania today.

Notes

The research for this chapter was conducted as part of a larger project that has been funded by National Science Foundation, IIE Fulbright, the University of North Carolina, and the University of Florida. A much earlier version of this essay was presented at the Amherst College for the Five Colleges' Culture and Medicine speakers' series. I thank those who attended that lecture for their thoughtful comments, particularly the careful reading given by Dr. Susan Shaw. I am also grateful for the feedback and critique by the discussants and participants of the 2002 American Anthropological Association Annual Meeting Healing Divides panel and those at the University of Pennsylvania Healing Divides workshop.

1. A German colony from 1891, Tanganyika was transferred at the end of the First World War to the British. It remained under British colonial administration until 1961.
2. In their landmark work on the history of science, *Leviathan and the Air-Pump*, Shapin and Schaffer (1985) have argued that solutions to problems of knowledge are also solutions to problems of social order.
3. This approach complements, even as it diverges from, Jean and John Comaroff's work (1997) concerning the encounter between the southern Tswana and the colonial evangelists of the British Nonconformist missionary societies. They argue that the friction between the missionaries' insistence on separating symbols and instruments and the Tswana's refusal of this separation opened "a breach in which a distinctly pragmatic African Christianity would take root" (333). In East Africa, such transformations can be traced in both Christianity and Islam. Here, however, I am following a different, albeit related, effect of the friction between missionaries and Africans in southeastern Tanzania—that is, the opening of a breach in which a distinctly scientific traditional medicine would take root.
4. As contemporary rereadings of colonial travel literature have illustrated, representational conventions often tell us more about the construction of the European "self" and the establishment of the "other"—whether that is the "African" or the "Orient"—than about how non-Europeans lived, worked, or

otherwise negotiated their worlds. For examples of postcolonial treatments of travel writing, see Clark (1999) and Pratt (1992).

5. Homi Bhabha reminds us that "[t]he question of the representation of difference is . . . always also a problem of authority" (1994, 89).

6. Although the transformations of this period are historically unique, and as we will see through the life of Leader Stirling, they are particularly relevant to national health care initiatives in Tanzania today, the fact of transformation is not unique to medicine. Feierman (1999) has noted that the relatively recent focus of Africanists on hybridity has, in aggregate, constructed colonialism as a primary or fundamental break in African history. Accounts abound of the emergence of precolonial/colonial hybrids or traditional/modern hybrids, but this discourse is rarely used to describe older historical transformations and encounters.

7. It was particularly at this moment that Stirling inhabited a space that Homi Bhabha calls the "in-between" in the *Location of Culture*. For Bhabha, those who creatively inhabit the uneasy spaces in between dominant categories and political positions can create the innovative identities that are most important to progressive politics. The play on multiple subject positions, which is more possible in these in-between spaces, serves as material for new and politically important tellings of the past and imaginings of the future.

8. See, for example, Griffin (1978), Keller (1985), Keller (1992), Merchant (1990), and Haraway (1989, 1991).

9. For examples of work concerning science and colonialism, see Prakash (1999) and MacLeod (2000). In relation to urban planning, see Mitchell (1988). In relation to issues of public health specifically, see Bashford (2003), Anderson (2001), and Hunt (1999).

10. The next and final sentence in this paragraph reads: "(Ujamaa villages have changed all that.)" *Ujamaa* was Nyerere's extensive restructuring project to bring social services and development to rural areas in Tanzania. The defining feature of *ujamaa* in the minds of many is the villagization policy, which attempted to move thousands of people from their homes and land into more condensed settlements around institutions such as hospitals and schools. This notion of broad-based socialist modernization insisted on a permanency and stability that stands in contrast to the mobility of the people in Stirling's description. Indeed, some have said that southern Tanzania was the most radically affected and changed by this period of government intervention (Liebenow 1971).

11. District Books are continuous logs kept by colonial officers stationed in each district. The Newala District Book (NDB) is available in the Tanzanian archive. It is a collection of observations, notes, comments, and occasionally an essay by district officers or by others who caught a district officer's attention. Entries in 1928 and the early 1940s are some of the most interesting in relation to agricultural practices in Newala.

12. Liebenow (1971).

13. Wolf (1982).

14. For explorations into nonhuman agency, see Barad (1999), Callon (1999), Latour (1988), and Latour (1999).

15. Jilek-Aall (1979).

16. Iliffe (1998).

17.   Iliffe (1979) sees the emergence of these movements as a response to the harsh punishment German colonial officers meted out against those accused of being witches and those who administered poison ordeals to detect witches. Ranger (1966) notes that eradication movements increased after the Maji Maji Rebellion (1905–1907) and that these movements also might be seen to resemble some aspects of the circulation of the medicines that were key to the rebellion. During the rebellion, which was the most profound resistance to foreign rule in Tanganyika, warriors from what had previously seemed to be unallied groups were mobilized through the circulation of medicinal water said to protect them from bullet wounds. By carrying "water" (Swahili, *maji*) from one group to another, experts referred to as *hongo* organized the widespread resistance against German rule. Witchcraft eradication movements also used medicine to organize social action.

8 Shifting Geographies of Suffering and Recovery: Traumatic Storytelling after Apartheid

Christopher J. Colvin

This chapter contributes to this volume's wider cartography of healing by examining the migrations of one particular therapeutic practice—traumatic storytelling—into, across, and beyond the South African landscape. It argues that traumatic storytelling—a therapeutically framed recounting of traumatic experiences—has developed in South Africa as a sometimes flexible but often surprisingly closed medical and political response to the various crises of post-apartheid South Africa. When traumatic storytelling was first introduced to South Africa, it was celebrated as more than a form of individual healing. It was supposed to transform the violent, long-suppressed history of apartheid into a new, shared national history. In the process, it was meant to reveal the forgotten common humanity of perpetrators, victims, and beneficiaries to each other. Through traumatic storytelling, South Africans were encouraged to challenge the old borders of race and construct new borders—temporal borders between past and present, social borders between the healed and the unhealed, and political borders between the new state and the old.

This chapter asks how and why a psychiatric discourse of trauma—put into practice in the form of traumatic storytelling—emigrated away from its spiritual homes in North America and Western Europe into places considerably less familiar with both the broad language of psychotherapy and the specific vocabulary of trauma. My first experience with trauma's inclination to travel was through media reports about South Africa's Truth and Reconciliation Commission (TRC).[1] I was struck by the way a psychotherapeutic discourse was interwoven with the more pronounced Christian and human rights discourses that framed the TRC. Phrases such as "the healing of a nation," "closure," "working through the past," "the trauma of apartheid," and "national catharsis" were part of an emerging political rhetoric about apartheid—and about the new political moment—that was rooted in a vocabulary of trauma and therapy.

In this chapter, I proceed roughly chronologically in tracking the movement and evolution of "traumatic storytelling" (defined below). I trace traumatic storytelling from its globalized origins and flourishing in the TRC to its encounters with local therapists, local victims, other modes of healing, and other parts of the country. I then follow traumatic storytelling—this time in new and unexpected forms—back into the global circuits of medicine and politics. In trying to account for its various routes and transformations, I consider a range of questions: Where does traumatic storytelling come from? Who embraces it and to what purposes? How is it controlled and transformed? How does it impact on local models of self, suffering, and recovery? What kinds of identities, boundaries, and affinities is it used to reinforce? The goal is to consider how traumatic storytelling both "works on" and "works for" patients and healers alike as it crosses and secures borders, old and new.

The Political Economy of Traumatic Storytelling

The traumatic storytelling examined here is grounded in the recently invented concepts of trauma and traumatic memory.[2] The many origins of trauma theory—as both an academic and wider cultural phenomenon—have been documented in a number of studies (Antze and Lambek 1996; Farrell 1998; Herman 1992; Leys 2000; Stone 1985; Young 1995). These historical surveys have highlighted the ways that the category "trauma" has been used to explain more and more about the personalities, behaviors, and emotional lives of individuals and societies (Hacking 1996). As trauma's explanatory capacity has expanded, so has its application; first to Vietnam veterans, then to victims of sexual and domestic abuse, to victims of all kinds of violence, to victims of natural disasters, and, finally, to those who have witnessed or even heard about traumatic events. Perhaps it is no surprise then that the use of this trauma discourse has also expanded geographically, first to the global epicenters of political violence, then to sites of natural disasters, and finally, increasingly, into the global everyday.

The particular variety of trauma discourse that emerged in South Africa was pieced together from various scientific, cultural, and political sources and then integrated with local contexts and concerns.[3] Rather than a wholesale importation of a psychological perspective, only those aspects of trauma theory relevant to framing and legitimizing local processes—such as the TRC—were borrowed into popular and political culture. Though South African psychologists have worked with trauma theory for a number of years (Lewis 1999; Swartz, Kerry, and Sandenbergh 2002), it was only through the TRC's embrace of "storytelling" about apartheid that the language and logic of trauma became widely understood. Victims who came to the TRC to testify and apply for reparations were asked to "tell their story" either to a statement taker or in a public, often televised hearing. Researchers and journalists flocked to South Africa in the mid-1990s to gather these stories and circulate them throughout the world.

NGOs that provided psychological support services counseled victims to come to individual or group therapy. Victims were frequently reminded that their own healing would flow only from the production of these stories of trauma, whether for the TRC, for therapists, for interested journalists, for concerned priests, or simply for friends and neighbors.

Encouraging victims to tell these stories tied into a larger postcolonial political discourse about the "right of recountability"—the rights of ordinary citizens to make public their private sufferings (Werbner 1998).[4] In South Africa, however, a victim's *right to* memory had a way of turning into a *demand for* memory by others, a kind of "memorial imperative" (Colvin 2001b). This demand for memory—whether from therapists, journalists, or politicians—was frequently justified in terms of the trauma discourse. At the TRC and elsewhere, victims were reminded that both personal and national recovery depended on this kind of narrative therapy. Testifying at the TRC thus became a way to heal one's self, to participate in a grand nation-building exercise, and to earn citizenship in the "New South Africa" (Wilson 2001).

The TRC's investment in trauma was a manifestation of the broader globalization of psychiatric knowledge about trauma (Breslau 2000). The global spread of traumatic storytelling, however, was facilitated not only through the field of mental health but also by the confessional narratives of soap operas, television dramas, and popular magazines. Trauma was, therefore, something that was "of the moment" in globalizing forms of popular culture, on middle-class talk shows, in magazines, and in movies. It was also, however, a discourse sustained by a range of political, institutional, and individual advocates. There is, for example, a large and growing network of trauma centers throughout the world (Summerfield 1999). Experts in trauma counseling are often flown to disaster sites around the globe at a moment's notice. Globalizing forms of trauma discourse and practice run parallel with globalizing forms of political intervention. Peacekeeping troops, conflict resolution experts, diplomats, scholars of democratization—all can often be found in the same hot zones of postconflict intervention as trauma counselors and debriefers. These experts at political and psychic reconstruction are inevitably accompanied by journalists and researchers who are eager to report on the latest forms of postconflict healing and eager to circulate the latest stories of traumatic violence. They reproduce these local traumatic stories and circulate them globally for the consumption of a diverse array of audiences.

Taken together, these diffuse actors, institutions, and interests—and the traumatic narratives of suffering that they produce, circulate, and consume—form a global "political economy of traumatic storytelling" (described in more detail in Colvin 2004). A constant stream of experts who fly to the next global hot spot to ask permission to record, interpret, and circulate victims' stories sustains this economy of narrative. In the process, victims' stories become commodified objects that move out into the wider world, producing new meanings and relationships in the process. Traumatic storytelling is the specific kind of labor required by this system of circulating stories and images. The term underscores three characteristic dimensions of this particular kind of storytelling. First, it is storytelling specifically about trauma. It is a kind of storytelling that does not easily admit the ambiguous or the mundane. Second, it is storytelling framed through the psychotherapeutic language of trauma. Third, it is a kind of storytelling that can itself be traumatizing to the teller.

How can we describe and account for the spread of this peculiar form of emotional and expressive labor and the social, political, and cultural effects it entails? Traumatic storytelling, like all healing discourses, brings together the problems of politics and healing.[5] When victims of apartheid were asked to "tell their stories" to various audiences, this process was always already cast both as political—as a way to perform the sign of the reconciled victim, to earn citizenship, or to write a new history—and as therapeutic—as individual and national healing. This dialectic between the therapeutic and the political is crucial for understanding the trajectory of traumatic storytelling in South Africa, since it was always through a combination of therapeutic imperatives and social and political demands that traumatic storytelling developed and traveled the routes it did in South Africa.

One of the major consequences of this market for narratives of suffering is that traumatic storytelling—which is promoted as both a healing and a political practice—has become *the* major way many victims negotiate their relationships with others. Maintaining a presence in the field of relations between the international community, their national government, civil society, the media, and the academy increasingly depends on their ability to produce and circulate engaging stories of suffering and recovery. How this came to be and how traumatic storytelling has been used and transformed in other contexts is the subject of the rest of this chapter.

The TRC as Medico-Political Art Form

Throughout much of the twentieth century, when South African psychologists weren't trying to diagnose "the African mind," they were busy serving the white population a familiar Euro-American brand of psychology (Bulhan 1993; Butchart 1998; Nicholas 1993). It was not in the context of middle-class psychology, however, that the concept of trauma first made its mark in South Africa. Traumatic storytelling first became part of the political and cultural lexicon on a national, public, and symbolic level, and the TRC provided its first and most prominent platform.

The TRC was an ambitious political project and its design and implementation was facilitated in large part by outside expertise, experience, and funding. Two high-profile international conferences were held in Cape Town to plan for the commission (Boraine, Levy, and Scheffer 1994; Boraine and Levy 1995). Numerous visiting academics and several local workshops and conferences were also part of the international effort to facilitate a truth commission (van der Merwe, DeWhirst, and Hamber 1999). Local NGOs banded together to create referral and lobbying networks such as the Mental Health Response to the TRC to manage the psychological aftermath of the TRC process (de Ridder 1997). Some of the most active members of these networks were the trauma clinics in Cape Town, Johannesburg, and Durban. A number of psychologists were also individually involved with the early planning, and several went on to become TRC commissioners. In the end, the religious and mental health communities—both foreign and local—provided the bulk of the input in the planning and implementation of the victim-centered aspects of the TRC (Lalu and Harris 1996, 33).

The influence of the mental health community is also evident in the TRC's own abundant use of psychological counselors. Several groups offered trauma counseling for those involved in the TRC (Pityana 1995). Debriefing counselors (informally called the "cry people") were available to witnesses before, during, and after hearings (TRC 1996a). The TRC also reported that a "team of therapists was brought in" to debrief the commissioners themselves on days of particularly gruesome testimony (TRC 1996a, Chapter 5).[6] Perpetrators of gross human rights violations even found occasion to put traumatic storytelling to use. Applying trauma theory to perpetrators was not difficult to effect theoretically,[7] but it generated a great deal of controversy in the commission and the media (Krog 1998, 76–78, 91–95).

In the meantime, victims were providing the enduring public face of traumatic storytelling. National and international networks broadcasted images of their traumatic memory-making around the world. Live public telecasts of the hearings each evening were a feature of South African life during much of the TRC. Prominent journalists and writers chronicled these spectacles of suffering, and documentary filmmakers seized on particularly dramatic visual moments of "catharsis" to tell about these stories. When each 30-minute bout of storytelling was over, the commissioners would often offer brief political and psychological interpretations, reframing specific details of victim testimony in terms of the broader moral messages of the commission (Ross 2003; Wilson 2001). Reluctant storytellers were reminded that healing could not come through silence. Successful storytellers were congratulated for having begun the difficult healing process and contributing to nation-building and reconciliation.

These were some of the most explicit and public mergers of the therapeutic and political vocabularies of trauma. In the process, a number of new borders were constructed and a number of old ones were challenged. Most important, traumatic storytelling was intended to craft a secure division between the past and the present. If anything, traumatic storytelling is about what is presumed to be over. It is a safe present speaking about an unsafe past. By facilitating the TRC process, the new state advertised itself as the inventor of this newly safe moment and distanced itself from its illegitimate predecessor (Wilson 2001). In identifying itself as a protector of human rights and the rule of law, the state also challenged the border that had long separated South Africa from the "community of nations" that respected modern liberal democratic values.

Truth-telling about the past was also supposed to enable the construction of clearer lines between victim, perpetrator, beneficiary, and witness by allowing individuals to stake claims on these particular social roles through their narrative labor. Those who refused to participate in the process enabled another kind of line to be drawn—between the reconciled and the unreconciled (Meister 1999). The process of traumatic storytelling was also a highly centralized one that was officially undertaken only in the presence of TRC staff or commissioners, the only ones who could certify individuals as "official" victims. This had the effect of creating boundaries of expert intervention where traumatic narratives—and the social roles and statuses they facilitated—could only be mediated by commissioners and TRC staff or, secondarily, by the journalists or therapists who followed up where the TRC left off.

The particular model of traumatic storytelling used at the TRC had the effect of reducing the meaning of "violation" to the violent, spectacular suffering of certain individuals rather than the structural and everyday violences visited on millions of individuals and communities during apartheid (Ross 2003). Suffering and healing became the province of the individual who had been subjected to the "extraordinary," to "trauma." Traumatic storytelling at the TRC became more public ritual than rigorous therapy or thoughtful historiography as it distilled experiences and packaged them into a "30-minute hour." In the process, it offered a way for a range of actors to promote new political messages—about reconciliation, about democracy, and about the evils of apartheid—and craft valuable new social identities—as long-suffering victims, repentant perpetrators, empathetic witnesses, or high-minded political leaders.

Trauma after the TRC

This ritualized model of traumatic storytelling persisted long after the TRC victim hearings ended. I first encountered it during fieldwork in late 1999, as public attention to traumatic storytelling had begun to fade. I wanted to follow the flow of therapeutic practice from the commission to the trauma clinic. At the beginning of my fieldwork, I had gathered many examples of the broad use of therapeutic language by the TRC but had little exposure to the work of trauma counseling as it was unfolding in South African consulting rooms. My first field site was the Cape Town Trauma Centre for Survivors of Violence and Torture, an NGO offering psychological counseling to victims of political and criminal violence. The Centre opened in 1993 in anticipation of the psychological needs of former political prisoners. Its therapeutic approach includes individual, group, couples, and family therapy. Additionally, some clients are assisted with "practical" problems such as filling out forms and obtaining referrals to social welfare and health organizations. Its therapeutic interventions are significantly informed by the psychiatric and psychotherapeutic trauma theories of the last twenty years (see van der Kolk, MacFarland, and Weisaeth 1995 for an overview).

I had hoped that the Trauma Centre would provide a rich source of clinical practice and discourse. However, its funding insecurities, its difficulty in convincing clients to commit to ongoing therapy, and the pressing nature of clients' survival needs meant that therapeutic relationships of any length or depth were hard to develop. In fact, in the Torture Project (a project within the Trauma Centre), there was very little in-depth counseling happening. Most of the clinical work consisted of intake and assessment, crisis interventions, referrals, a few inconsistently attended counseling sessions, and lots and lots of social work.

If there wasn't much counseling happening, there were certainly many foreign visitors. The Trauma Centre's funders are almost exclusively intergovernmental organizations, foreign churches, and human rights and psychological support organizations in Europe and the United States. These funders would frequently travel to Cape Town to see how their money was being spent. Some of them were setting up similar trauma programs in other countries and were seeking advice on how to translate the Trauma Centre's work into other contexts. The Trauma Centre is also a hub for foreign psychologists, researchers, and journalists. All of these people came to visit the Trauma Centre to investigate its therapeutic work. More importantly, though, most of them also came to meet and spend time with "victims." The victims they were interested in were members of the Khulumani (Speak Out!) Support Group, which had begun as an effort by the Torture Project and some local victim advocates to address the material, social, and psychological needs of victims after the TRC. The group eventually separated from the Trauma Centre and established itself as an independent victim advocacy and support group, though they continue to meet with the Centre in what are called the "monthly meetings."

From the beginning, these monthly meetings have been divided into two parts. The first half of the meeting is devoted to "advocacy" issues and the second half is reserved for "storytelling." The storytelling section has been less a structured psychological intervention and more an informal chance to tell stories of suffering to people who have had similar experiences. Trauma Centre staff facilitate these storytelling sessions. For a long time, the traumatic storytelling work during these monthly meetings resembled the TRC hearings: the same short block of time for narration, the same narrow focus on traumatic events during apartheid, the same language of trauma, working through, and catharsis.

As the hype around the TRC began to fade, though, both group members and therapists began experimenting with these sessions, trying to encourage more interaction between people (rather than just rote storytelling) and trying to incorporate nontraumatic aspects of people's pasts into their narratives. The standard models of trauma therapy have proven unsuited to the group for a number of reasons. In particular, the TRC-inspired model of traumatic storytelling focused on exceptional acts of violence and terror experienced by a relative few. It was principally monological—a lone victim speaking to the commission, the cameras, and the nation. And it cast the apartheid era as the primary source of contemporary suffering, making critiques of the current moment difficult to mount. Khulumani and the Trauma Centre tried to respond to these limitations by incorporating the present, the mundane, and the communal into its narrative strategies.

The ability to change and make use of traumatic storytelling has not been the same, however, for group members and for the therapists. Storytelling has been useful to group members on a number of levels. It has facilitated the emergence of a strong group identity. Since many in the group are not victims of "gross violations" of human rights, traumatic storytelling has expanded the boundaries of victimhood and increasingly located suffering in the social, the structural, and the everyday. It has reinforced the illegitimacy of the apartheid state and clarified for group members the boundaries between victim, perpetrator, and beneficiary. It has also become a means of "resource mobilization"—as it often was at the TRC—for victims who seek compensation, services, and recognition of their suffering.

The therapists, however, often have found themselves reinforcing contrasting meanings and messages. Their theoretical perspectives, rooted in conventional trauma theory, made it difficult for them to incorporate present-day, structural forms of suffering into their interventions, despite their awareness that these continuing violences were affecting the mental health of group members. The line between past and present also remained central to their work even though group members were constantly arguing for the continuing effects of the past in the present. They confronted a similar difficulty in integrating, as they saw it, the distinct problems of material suffering and psychological suffering. They spoke constantly about the interplay between the two, but their therapeutic approach was always rooted in the psychological and they maintained a strict separation between different domains of care—psychological, spiritual, material, social, and political. This meant that their interventions also tended to reinforce the tense border between expert healer and novice patient that is part of the social character of much psychology. Though they challenged the simplistic models of narrative therapy circulated through the TRC, they often found themselves at odds with the ways in which group members were seeking to use the memory work of storytelling.

After the TRC, then, we see many of the same actors and institutions involved in promoting and reshaping traumatic storytelling. In this new post-TRC context, however, the purposes to which traumatic storytelling was put to use expanded considerably. Outside the narrow framework of the TRC, victims had much more range of motion in trying to use traumatic storytelling to enlarge what it means to be a victim and criticize the lack of change in their lives since the end of apartheid. For therapists, traumatic storytelling provided an ongoing source of legitimacy for their own work and an ongoing source of funding from overseas agencies. They tried to adapt traumatic storytelling in ways that were more responsive to the victims they were working with but found themselves constrained by disciplinary boundaries and the priorities of funders. Those active in the global political economy of traumatic storytelling during the TRC remained active afterward, and the raw material of these traumatic narratives continued to sustain their work, whether academic, religious, therapeutic, or political.

Trauma, Nerves, *Satani,* and the Ancestors

So far in this story, traumatic storytelling has made its way from various psychologists, NGOs, and researchers to the TRC, the Trauma Centre, and on to Khulumani. In the process, parts of it were selectively adopted and transformed to better meet the needs and interests of each particular context. From inside the Trauma Centre, though, it began to feel like everyone in South Africa was talking about trauma. I was reminded about a wider, more complex reality, however, by a fellow anthropologist, Hayley MacGregor, who was doing fieldwork at a local public hospital on the experiences and understandings of mental distress among local township residents (MacGregor 2002).

Her work was focusing on one of the local terms of distress, *i-nevs,* or "nerves," a common idiom worldwide for a wide variety of what biomedicine would identify as mental and physical ailments. As she was describing the semantic flexibility of the nerves concept and its ability to account for many kinds of illness, I realized that I had never heard the word "*i-nevs*" in the whole time I had worked with the Trauma Centre and Khulumani—at that point around ten months. Many of the problems of Khulumani members could certainly have been captured in this language of nerves. It was clear, though, that they employed a language of trauma instead.

Likewise, MacGregor reported that she had rarely heard psychiatric patients at the public hospital speak about "trauma" in the same way Khulumani members did. I asked some Khulumani members about the nerves concept and they all agreed that they were suffering from nerves. I asked if nerves were related to "trauma" and they replied that sometimes memories of trauma caused their nerves to "rise." They explained that many things could make one's nerves rise—trauma, witchcraft, trouble with family or friends, or physical diseases. I asked why they never spoke of "nerves" at the Trauma Centre. Most of them responded that their therapists were interested in trauma—nerves, they said, interested the doctors.

Another anthropologist, Jennifer Badstuebner, noted that in her work on witchcraft in a Cape Town township, she had seen a similar division between talk of nerves and talk of witchcraft. Problems that at the hospital might have been described as "having nerves" were often identified to her as problems of bewitchment. She argued that distress presented in one domain would be framed in terms appropriate to that domain. This tacking back and forth between different therapeutic frameworks is not an unusual phenomenon. Medical anthropology has long recognized that the use of multiple explanatory models is neither uncommon nor necessarily inconsistent. Here, traumatic storytelling was clearly one therapeutic option among many. What is striking, however, is its very specific geographic and demographic profile. In these cases, victims lived in the townships but only spoke about trauma with professionals who worked and lived in the city center.[8] The clear divide in therapeutic vocabulary highlighted the even starker divisions between the townships and the city center.

This isn't a simple case of medical pluralism, however, with easily delineated discourses and practices of healing that the patient can choose from rationally or instrumentally. MacGregor noted later that many patients she saw spoke freely of witchcraft as an underlying or aggravating cause. Likewise, Badstuebner (2003) has written of the dramatic tales of witchcraft that took place in a church she visited during her fieldwork. And in fact, when I spent time with Khulumani members at the Trauma Centre, I began to recognize talk of nerves when members arrived early for meetings and were chatting. I also heard them speak about trauma to their family and community when I visited their homes in the townships. It is clear that all four of these therapeutic perspectives inter-penetrated in different ways and were not seen to necessarily contradict, or even be distinct from, one another.

That said, it is interesting that while talk of witches, *Satani* (Satan), nerves, and trauma can freely combine in many contexts, within the institutional boundaries of the Trauma Centre, trauma talk held an almost exclusive sway. The institutional context and the social relationships that had been established between therapist and client served to make talk of other models of suffering somehow out of bounds. It wasn't that therapists mocked alternative theories of distress or intentionally regulated the borders of their own practice. They even recognized that Christian spirituality, beliefs in witchcraft, and indigenous terms for physical distress were important in understanding and intervening in mental health. Nonetheless, trauma remained as the nearly exclusive language at the Trauma Centre.

So why the exclusivity? Why the closure of the discourse of trauma? The apparent policing of its boundaries? It is unlikely that traumatic storytelling is somehow too unfamiliar, too "Western" for local incorporation. Healing prac-tices have proven greatly—though not infinitely—inventive in their incorpora-tion of the unfamiliar. I consider this question in more detail in the final section of this chapter, but for now, one observation. The one thing that sets traumatic storytelling apart from these other therapeutic modalities is that it is the only intervention that confers a politically valuable identity on sufferers. It is the only one that distinguishes certain traumatized individuals and their claims for rec-ognition from the rest of the suffering poor who populate post-apartheid South Africa. Perhaps it is not to anyone's advantage to confuse the issue by mention-ing witchcraft, divine intervention, or nerves in a context so rich with potential to confer recognition and even compensation to victims of political violence. Similarly, those providing trauma counseling also benefit by being identified with this unique and politically valued intervention. The Trauma Centre enjoys a public profile and respect unmatched by any primary care provider, religious outreach project, or traditional healer that also works with victims of violence.

From City to Suburb and Township

If the politicized language of trauma is not as evident in the townships or hospitals as it is the Trauma Centre, the trauma discourse is nonetheless making its way into public health facilities, but this time through a different route. MacGregor mentioned that the one place she had come across descriptions of trauma was through posters in local hospitals that described post-traumatic stress disorder (PTSD) and listed its primary symptoms. Patients were also slowly becoming aware of the fact that a diagnosis of PTSD might qualify them for a disability grant. The language of trauma is also establishing itself in the private health care system in response to the effects of criminal violence. Several popular handbooks dealing with trauma in the South African context have been published (Lewis 1999; Swartz, Kerry, and Sandenbergh 2002). Several communities in the suburbs of Cape Town are setting up trauma rooms at local police stations to serve victims of violent crime. Even advertising circulars for department store credit cards highlight the provision of 24-hour trauma counseling as a benefit of membership.

So the trauma discourse is being brought into the public and private health systems and moving closer to the lives of everyday people, but this time in a different form. Where the language of trauma began its life in the TRC as a part of a political language of complaint among victims of apartheid, it has migrated to the townships as part of a wider vocabulary of public health. And in the middle-class suburbs, the trauma discourse is shifting away from the political critique of apartheid and tapping into a newer political discourse about the post-apartheid rise of crime in South Africa.

Talk in the suburbs about trauma is usually tied up in a broader political argument about the "chaotic" state of affairs since apartheid ended and the heightened sense of vulnerability middle-class residents feel. Talk about trauma in the townships also highlights the rise of violent crime, but the critique of crime in the townships is usually linked to the broad historical sweep of apartheid. Where suburban trauma talk refers to the *new* traumas of the post-apartheid moment, township trauma talk connects new traumas with *old* ones and asserts, contrary to the TRC, that apartheid is not over.

It is significant that as it has moved from political violence to criminal violence, from the city to the suburb and township, the practice of public traumatic storytelling has been downplayed. Where victims of political violence are encouraged to publicly narrate their stories of suffering, victims of criminal violence are more often than not simply put on antidepressants. In moving beyond political violence, traumatic storytelling seems to have lost its narrative impulse and become more of a psychiatric problem for biomedicine than a psychological and political problem of interest to therapists, journalists, and politicians. It still operates as an avenue of political complaint (against the lingering crimes of apartheid or the new crimes of democratic South Africa), but its public narrative dimension has diminished.

The Gospel of *i-Trauma*

The embrace of traumatic storytelling by the TRC, the Trauma Centre and Khulumani, and the public and private health systems has been a largely urban phenomenon. In fact, most of the NGOs offering trauma-related services are located in South Africa's three major cities—Cape Town, Durban, and Johannesburg. These organizations have very little presence in the rural areas, where more than half of the South African population lives. Early in my fieldwork, the Trauma Centre and Khulumani decided that they wanted to undertake rural outreach to this underserved population. Both groups painted a grim picture of desperately poor communities suffering without access to their services. A great deal of urgency, even nostalgia, was invested in the idea of rural outreach.

On my first trip to the countryside, I accompanied three Khulumani members who were recruiting rural members for the Cape Town group. One of the Khulumani members, Monwabisi, spoke at length to people about Khulumani and the importance of counseling. He told me that this recruiting trip was a chance to spread the "gospel of Khulumani" but that Khulumani could not help people with all of their psychological problems. For that, the "gospel of *i-trauma*" was necessary. Fortunately, I did not advertise my connection with the Trauma Centre during this trip. Hostile and frustrated comments about the Centre soon bubbled to the surface. Unbeknown to me, the Centre had already tried to set up satellite clinics in this area several times and the few efforts they had put together had failed. It had not committed the energy and resources necessary to make these outreach efforts successful. Each time they closed a satellite clinic, local residents grew more resentful and more confused about what the Centre was trying to do in their community. A number of previous victim advocacy groups from Cape Town had also tried to recruit members from these areas with similar results. People in these communities felt burned by both of these groups, and the Khulumani members had a rough time trying to prove their sincerity and trustworthiness.

Despite Monwabisi's advocacy of counseling and traumatic storytelling among the rural populace, the "gospel of *i-trauma*" never took hold in the places we visited. Few trauma-oriented NGOs in South Africa have developed sustained programs of trauma counseling outside cities. The difficulty in extending traumatic storytelling to rural areas is mirrored in the difficulties trauma organizations have had in other countries in southern Africa. Most of these countries might be expected to be natural markets for traumatic storytelling in both its more politicized and its more medicalized forms. For the most part, though, this has not happened. Several of these countries—Namibia and Mozambique in particular—have frequently been singled out for their emphasis on a kind of postconflict *silence* rather than the public purging of emotion that was the rule in South Africa (Boswall 1999; Honwana 1999; Pakleppa 1999).

Earlier, I noted the possible reasons for the closure of the trauma discourse. Here one might ask why traumatic storytelling failed to take hold in the rural areas and in countries beyond the borders of South Africa. Cultural differences could be a factor. Those working in Mozambique and Namibia, for example, have argued that the confessional and verbal character of traumatic storytelling is foreign to some cultural notions of the proper relationships between self, suffering, and recovery. Certainly traumatic storytelling's public airing of what some might consider private, if not shameful, experiences and feelings chafes even the urbanized residents in Cape Town. Traumatic storytelling may be very familiar to most South Africans through the globalized television viewing and magazine reading they do, but as a local practice, it has very few precedents. "Testimony" at churches and anti-apartheid speech-making and literature are perhaps the closest preexisting modes of traumatic narrative, but these forms of storytelling took place, and continue to take place, in very different contexts and with very different end goals.

Perhaps the rural areas simply remain isolated to a large degree from the public, political discourses of traumatic storytelling and from the fruits of this discourse. And perhaps there are not enough resources for the urban advocates of traumatic storytelling to bring their message of narrative redemption to the vast rural landscape. Perhaps the romance of rural outreach is just that for most—a romance, easily undermined by the significant difficulties of work in these areas. Whatever the range of possible reasons, however, traumatic storytelling, in its various permutations, has primarily been an urban South African phenomenon.

The Return of the Repressed, or the Empire Narrates Back

Far from conquering the political or therapeutic imaginations of southern Africans, traumatic storytelling seems to have traveled a much more restricted route. In fact, even in the heartlands of traumatic storytelling, it has not had the easiest time. For example, the split between the Trauma Centre and Khulumani was largely predicated on the feeling among Khulumani members that traumatic storytelling was increasingly unable to address their needs. Their fight with the government over the delay in reparations payments energized them. Some members of Khulumani came to see the Trauma Centre as a politically conservative collection of individuals who, though well-intentioned, were only interested in providing a narrow kind of medical treatment rather than a broadly imagined psychological, social, and political intervention. One member said,

> They just want us to be victims and tell our stories so they can help us. I am sick of telling my story. It makes them feel good to show that they are helping us. They don't really want to change things and what good does telling our stories over and over and over do? They are just white professionals who want to keep their jobs.

In this context, traumatic storytelling came to be seen as a less relevant and potentially distracting practice if not an activity in opposition to the requirements of justice and reconciliation. Another member said,

> We will decide now when and how we want the storytelling, but we can't let it interfere with our work. Yes, storytelling is important, but let's not get so stuck on it. . . . We can't forget our real mission . . . reparations.

However, even as the group was moving away from the Trauma Centre and its therapeutic approach to storytelling, it was also trying to redeploy traumatic storytelling as an instrument and expression of political discontent. This time, however, they wanted the production of traumatic narratives to be on their own terms.

Eight months after Khulumani separated from the Trauma Centre, the group organized a two-day conference intended to force the government to enter into discussions around the long-awaited reparations policy. At a press conference a week before the meeting, Khulumani told reporters that their members would be "telling their stories" at the meeting but that the press would not be allowed to interview or otherwise "harass" them. A two-page document providing names and short biographical details of these victims would be circulated to journalists who wanted to write about them, but these synopses would be available only at the end of the conference and only to those who attended both days of meetings.

The reporters in attendance seemed a bit surprised but went along with the arrangements. At the conference, Khulumani members did get up and tell their stories. The photojournalists duly captured these dramatic scenes and the stories of these victims began appearing in the newspapers. Khulumani members offered these stories as a sign of the continuing suffering of its members. They emphasized this kind of storytelling as evidence of traumatic stress and psychological illness and celebrated the Trauma Centre for its work in helping some of its members. It is ironic that this recognition of the value of therapy occurred at a moment when Khulumani was perhaps the most estranged from the Trauma Centre in terms of daily interactions and interpersonal tensions.

Rather than emphasizing the specific medical histories and outcomes of individuals, though, traumatic storytelling here was presented as a more general sign of medico-political distress. Khulumani deployed the medicalized language of trauma, but this time with their own, very specific political point to make. Safely out of the orbit of the Trauma Centre, they now embraced the medical language of trauma—and the legitimizing effects of this scientific discourse—and presented their members as angry, still-suffering victims of both medical and political dis-ease. They reminded their audience about the failure of trauma therapy and other outside interventions to address the full range of their concerns.

Reparations are usually figured by Khulumani as the missing piece of the therapeutic puzzle for victims. Their fight for reparations has found them traveling back over the same international routes that brought them traumatic storytelling. Where foreign human rights NGOs, governments, and psychologists brought much of the model of traumatic storytelling to South Africa, Khulumani is now traveling back to Europe and the United States and talking with these same NGOs and government agencies. This time, however, the conversation is about reparations. The language of trauma still figures prominently in these negotiations, but it is now mobilized for the fight for reparations. They are meeting with representatives of these foreign agencies, distributing documentary films, and traveling to Europe not as a way of demanding more psycho-therapeutic services but as a way to seek financial and symbolic compensation for their suffering. The recent suits filed against American, European, and South African companies for apartheid-related reparations are certain to use a thera-peutic discourse of (and expert witnesses in) trauma to identify and legitimize the harms being claimed in court. The psychotherapeutic has thus become more of a medical means to a range of legal and political ends than the end in itself the TRC had originally envisioned.

Closure

As a range of actors—including victims, therapists, doctors, politicians, academics, and journalists—have moved traumatic storytelling across the vari-ous landscapes of South Africa and beyond, they have reinforced and reshaped old borders and helped create new borders between people, places, ideas, and moments in time. In the process, they have transformed traumatic storytelling. Like any discourse, traumatic storytelling is not infinitely flexible. It retains its biomedical ancestry and its tendency to medicalize and pathologize. And its usefulness in various political projects—whether it be "nation-building" or vic-tim protest—means that it is always bound up in the political as much as the therapeutic. The circuitous path traumatic storytelling has traced through South Africa reveals that it is sufficiently plastic to be more than a simple imposition of a rigid, outside, "Western" therapy onto a "local" context. It has, in the words of this volume's editors, "creatively [produced] healing ideologies and practices that assign order and meaning in profound and unexpected ways."

However, there is a peculiar inflexibility to traumatic storytelling as well. This intractability of traumatic storytelling, its closure against integration into local idioms of distress, was raised by Richard Werbner in his comments on the conference version of this chapter. Though I have traced a number of ways that traumatic storytelling has been reshaped by different actors, the fact remains that it hasn't been integrated into South African culture in the ways other West-ern medical technologies have been. Furthermore, the lack of trauma talk in the townships, in the country, and the antagonism to some modes of trauma talk in Khulumani suggests that those trying to promote traumatic storytelling have not been too successful in importing and adapting this practice to the South African context.

Why might this be? Does traumatic storytelling not resonate sufficiently with local generative principles? Would the closure of the trauma discourse pro-vide a counterexample to Megan Vaughn's contention that African communities have always been remarkably inventive in their adaptations of outside healing systems? In some places, people have deployed traumatic storytelling with the kind of innovation and creativity necessary for successful adaptation to the lo-cal. In others, it has fallen flat. Why? In considering why a particular discourse does or doesn't change, we can ask about local incentives to incorporate and adapt and we can also examine the external forces that might be invested in keeping a discourse stable within its original boundaries.

I have previously pointed to both the local history of psychological knowledge and practice and the dramatic influx of psychological expertise during the TRC. The labeling of postconflict crises as psychological problems—rather than (also) political, social, economic, or moral problems—is certainly convenient for intervening peacekeeping nations that want to promote peaceful transitions toward democracy but do not want to get involved in the lingering structural difficulties of postconflict societies. Recasting the wide-ranging effects of violence as primarily psychological invites a limited and scientific response to suffering —an intervention with an exit strategy. This is just as true for the new state. Trauma therapy and its focus on the management of individual emotion—in particular, emotions of depression, anxiety, and revenge—resonate with the wider South African nation-building discourse of restorative justice, "*ubuntu*" (an "African" form of humanism), and reconciliation. This, in effect, limits the state's burden to respond more broadly to the structural and everyday suffering of these citizens.

Likewise, the political usefulness of traumatic storytelling in negotiating the meaning of history in the new nation is well documented. Historiography can serve both to foster a sense of national unity and to legitimize the new state as the rightful provider for and representative of the people (Wilson 2001). History—whether triumphalist or traumatic—not only unifies and legitimizes but also provides a moral education to its public. The sight of weeping victims at the TRC, the shocking contents of their traumatic narratives, and the rabbinical interpretations offered by the commissioners were lessons to the public (and to a skeptical world) about the past and about the core values of the new state and society. In contexts outside the TRC, traumatic storytelling provided an opportunity for healers and patients alike to comment on the meaning of the past. Trauma Centre therapists claimed that they could help victims understand their traumatic pasts. Victims, on the other hand, countered that the version of the past the Trauma Centre was promoting was not their past but their present. A similar contradiction existed between suburban trauma talk that used trauma to speak about the new traumas of contemporary violence and township trauma talk that linked the present with the past.

We might look to institutional agendas as well. There is quite an active trauma industry at work in disaster-prone areas of the world, and self-perpetuation might be part of the reason for the inflexibility of the trauma discourse. Certainly the Trauma Centre, which defines itself through the provision of a very specific service to a narrow range of individuals, finds it difficult to not find trauma everywhere it looks. The vigorous expansion across the globe of concepts of trauma is facilitated by the idealistic individuals and institutions that have taken up the challenge to attend to the traumatized. Moreover, traumatic storytelling is most often deployed by these organizations as a kind of expert process in need of expert management and intervention, something that closes rather than opens the discourse and establishes hierarchical social relationships of expert and patient.

Individual Trauma Centre therapists, despite their awareness of Khulumani's critiques of traumatic storytelling, found it very difficult to adapt their theory and practice. Perhaps this is partly because it is just too difficult to quickly adapt psychological theories that have risen out of centuries of social and cultural development to non-Western postcolonial contexts. In addition, the influence of funders had a significant impact on practice at the Trauma Centre. These funders were interested in providing torture victims, former political prisoners, and other glamorous victims of gross human rights violations with the redeeming technologies of trauma therapy. Despite the Trauma Centre's creative efforts to justify their work with the broad membership of Khulumani as work with torture victims, their funding framework never provided serious room for creativity and innovation. This raises a question about how much agency individual healers can assert within the context of broader discursive, economic, and political realities. The inability of the Trauma Centre to meaningfully change much of its intervention despite a thorough awareness of the difficulties with its approach and a commitment to improving its services speaks to the broader structures, interests, and agendas that individual healers or institutions may be bound up in.

Khulumani adapted traumatic storytelling to its own ends and sought to capitalize on the scientific language of trauma and its ability to legitimate victim identities. At the same time, the group criticized the practice of trauma therapy as conservative hand-wringing on the part of guilty white South Africans. They transformed the trauma discourse into an instrument of their fight for reparations and managed at the same time to extricate themselves from what they felt was the less-than-useful work of therapy at the Trauma Centre. What they did not do, however, was significantly transform or integrate traumatic storytelling into other local modes of relief or expression, whether religious, political, or sociocultural. They reproduced the form and sign of traumatic storytelling even as they critiqued it, and they did not do very much to make it over into something new.

Khulumani's use of traumatic storytelling and the embrace of the trauma discourse in suburban complaints about crime demonstrate that it is a practice that can be deployed by patient and healer alike. This does not contradict the argument about the role of expertise in policing the borders of traumatic storytelling. Any particular discourse is not in itself an "expert discourse" or a "folk discourse." Whether or not the social relationships of expertise prevail within the particular practice of a discourse depends on the context in which it is put to use. Within the bounds of the Trauma Centre and the TRC, traumatic storytelling functioned as an expert discourse that reproduced power relationships between the governing and the governed, between healer and the healed. But in the suburbs, where middle-class egalitarianism is the rule, traumatic storytelling was deployed with ease by nonexperts. Similarly, in the protest work of

Khulumani, though power differences continued to prevail, members were able through their confrontation and resistance to these differences to deploy traumatic storytelling to their own ends and undo the tendency of this scientific language to privilege the educated expert over the uneducated patient.

Despite the ways traumatic storytelling has been transformed as it has moved through the South African landscape, despite its enthusiastic reception in the suburbs and its redeployment by victims as a new kind of medico-political critique, it remains a bit of a puzzle. Perhaps in its deep concern with the dramatic and individuated violences often labeled as trauma, it simply misses much of what happens every day in South Africa. Any broad and successful therapeutic framework, any theodicy of self, suffering, and recovery, needs to be able to capture a significant portion of the experiences of the ordinary. Perhaps at the end of the day, in order to work against the closure that seems to rope traumatic storytelling off from other therapeutic modes and practices, its practitioners may need to reinvent traumatic storytelling as a science of the ordinary before it can speak to the endemic traumas of the southern African region.

Notes

None of this work would have been possible without the support and trust of the members of Khulumani and the Trauma Centre. I am also grateful to Natalie Leon and Hayley MacGregor for their helpful comments on this essay. The research was funded by grants from the Academy for Educational Development, the Institute for the Study of World Politics, and the Anthropology Department of the University of Virginia. Completion of this essay was supported by the Center for Comparative Literature and Society at Columbia University.

1. The TRC was set up after the 1994 democratic elections to provide victims of "gross human rights violations" a chance to testify to their sufferings under apartheid and give perpetrators of violations the opportunity to confess and apply for amnesty for their crimes. See Wilson (2001) and Ross (2003) for a fuller description.
2. Though many of those who write about trauma look to "shell-shock," "railway spine," or even to the ancient tales of Gilgamesh and Homer's *Iliad* to establish the deep historicity of "trauma" (Herman 1992; Parry-Jones and Parry-Jones 1994; Shay 1994), I am concerned here with the recent elaboration of a distinct psychiatric discourse of trauma (see Young 1995 on the features of the discourse and on the term "inventing").
3. See Colvin 2001a for an account of the specific similarities and differences.
4. Note, however, that unlike many cases of popular countermemory that assert Werbner's "right of recountability" against a violent state that silences, in this case, the TRC and the government were the main proponents of this right. The function of this right in the political calculus of post-apartheid memory is, therefore, quite different.

5. The relationship between the medical and the political is an old debate and will not be rehearsed here. See Janzen (2001) for a useful elaboration of this issue.
6. The lawyers and the audience at the hearings were also eligible for counseling, because they, like the commissioners, might be victims of "secondary victimization" (Hamber 1997, 14). This therapeutic ethic was even extended to those not found to be victims of gross human rights violations, since failing to qualify for victim status was understood to be in itself a traumatizing event (TRC 1996b).
7. The recent model of traumatic stress in fact derives from the experiences of Vietnam War veterans, many of whom were diagnosed with PTSD after having committed or witnessed acts of violence.
8. The Trauma Centre is located near the center of Cape Town, at least fifteen to twenty miles from where most of its clients live.

Afterword: Ethnographic Regions—Healing, Power, and History

Steven Feierman

The idea of the border is one anthropologists have meditated on since the founding of the field in its early-twentieth-century version. It is, after all, impossible to imagine the world through the eyes of people living in another culture unless one explores their ways of classifying the natural world—dividing north from south (or dividing directions in some other way), zenith from nadir, life from death, winter from spring, and our people from others (whoever "we" are). Between each category and each other the anthropologist necessarily finds a boundary. How else to establish the fact of separation? For Durkheim and Mauss, writing in the first decade of the twentieth century, each of the major boundaries in the observed and imagined worlds of nature or the spirits was also at the same time a line of separation in the social world, for example between the people we marry and those we don't or between one descent group and another (1903/1963). Arnold van Gennep, writing in the same decade, showed the relationship between movement across territorial borders and movements between states of being—from stranger to homeperson, from secular to sacred, or from sexually immature person to adult (1908/1960). Whether in rites of passage or in movements across the landscape, a crucial culturally charged moment came at the point of transition, on the threshold (the *limen*). Victor Turner's work, more than half a century later, explored the power of liminality, the boundary state, betwixt and between, where (for a moment) people could experience life as neither child nor adult, neither man nor woman, and yet endowed with the fruitful power of the boundary (1967, 93–111).

The authors of the present volume return to boundary work but in a very different spirit from Durkheim, or Mauss, or van Gennep, or even from Turner. In the 1960s, stable zones of citizenship and culture seemed clear and the idea of categories seemed unproblematic. But liminal zones—regions of unstable meaning, uncertain citizenship, and symbolic power—called for explanation. Now forty years later, borders, even legally fixed national borders, seem relative and artifactual (that is, arbitrary products of human activity; Hannerz 1997), washed away by global flows in full flood, flows that leave us only with what Appadurai has called "scapes"—fluid, rough, dynamically evolving divisions of the world's landscapes—ethnoscapes, or technoscapes, or financescapes, and so on (1997). Where earlier generations of thinkers found it necessary to explain the characteristics of an unstable and fertile border region between categories, between nations, or between phases of ritual action, the authors of this volume know the world of fertile instability in their bones (and acknowledge it in their writings) but find it problematic that people in motion are able to construct worlds in which the idea of a clear separation remains—that the border does not dissolve completely into indeterminacy but remains a border, with two sides, each with its own characteristics. In a fluid world, the idea of the boundary does not become irrelevant but remains a source of power.

The essays in this book, taken as a group, find a creative solution to the problem of boundedness and flow in the cultures of healing by exploring the issues within a loosely defined ethnographic region. In doing so they have opened up questions about the contribution of comparative ethnography within a supralocal, transnational region that is, in spite of its openness, unmistakably situated on the African continent. The region they define has a powerfully important set of characteristics that cannot be found anywhere else in the world: to say that it is transnational is not to say that it lacks a hugely important sense of place.

There are strong precedents for using comparative anthropological methods within regions larger than local societies but smaller than continents and for defining those regions in ways that are not constrained by the boundaries of a colony or of a nation-state. In the 1950s, some of the most sophisticated anthropologists in the United States and Britain were searching for ways to make valid comparisons across cultures and decided that regional studies were a way to do this, through the method of "controlled comparison." By holding many shared environmental elements constant and by dealing with languages and cultural practices that were closely related to one another within a region, the anthropologists were able to reason more clearly about the nature of pattern and variation. Fred Eggan and Isaac Schapera both advocated controlled comparison. Eggan wrote that his "own preference is for the utilization of the comparative method on a smaller scale and with as much control over the frame of comparison as it is possible to secure. It has seemed natural to utilize regions of relatively homogeneous cultures or to work with social or cultural types, and to further control the ecology and historical factors so far as it is possible to do so" (Eggan 1954, 747; Schapera 1953). Evans-Pritchard argued for much the same thing but then thought that the method might potentially be weak because it would be "more likely to lead to historical conclusions than laws of the natural science type which anthropologists have aimed at establishing" (1963, 21).[1] Today, of course, anthropologists are deeply interested in just the sort of interpretive, historically contextualized studies produced by controlled comparison. And in fact some of the richest bodies of ethnographic research that have been produced in Africa have come from anthropologists working intensively on related problems within a region, with strong attention to time and place. This was certainly the case in central Africa in the work of anthropologists associated with the Rhodes-Livingstone Institute and Manchester University (Schumaker 2001).

Regional studies at the present moment, half a century later, look quite different, of course, with their fuller attention to history and to global flows.

It is possible to explain what makes southeast Africa a region in several different ways. First, the African people of the region have been forced to respond to the harsh challenges of colonial rule in a form that here (even more than in many other parts of Africa) was violent, racialized, and economically exploitative. One reason the region's healing cultures share a common style is that they have all had to respond to these extreme challenges. A second source of commonality stems from shared language and history, going back deeply into the region's precolonial past. The different languages of southeast Africa are closely related to one another, and along with this common linguistic heritage comes a shared heritage in the healing ideas and practices that are encoded in language. Third, and finally, the region's healing practices share many elements because of the process of circulation: people have always learned from one another across cultural boundaries, and they still do so today, as many of this book's contributions demonstrate.

First we look at the colonial challenges the region faced. The regimes of racial rule in southeast Africa since the late nineteenth century (and in some places earlier) subjected people to kinds of psychic and physical violence that had deep similarities across many local African societies and led to profound needs for healing. In some places, Africans served in the police and formed irregular armies to help with the conquest of their own region. This was the case with the Chikunda—the ethnic category adopted by the men who served as enforcers under the Portuguese (Isaacman 2004). In South Africa and in all the colonies, white rule came only after a period of violent conquest, often leading to a period of disruption and upheaval that had serious consequences for the health of the people. The conquest of Zimbabwe, for example, was followed by a period of famine, locusts, and disease. A panzootic wiped out a large percentage of the cattle herds (Ranger 1967, 148; Iliffe 1990, Chapter 3). Southern Tanzania suffered huge population losses in the first decade of the twentieth century (that is, the second decade of colonial rule).

Because conquest came in the form of a crisis of health and survival, it had a profound effect in shaping the region's healing landscapes. It meant that prominent healers and spirit mediums, who were the appropriate people to respond to crises of health, played a major role in responding to colonial disruption. They were the local intellectuals who helped people think through the meaning of this new and dangerous era. The Isaacmans have written about the importance of spirit mediums in Mozambican resistance movements of the late nineteenth and early twentieth centuries. And in Zimbabwe, the names of Nehanda and Kagubi, two famous mediums during the uprising of 1896–1897, are still known today. They are the subjects of plays and popular political songs (Isaacman and Isaacman 1976; Ranger 1967; Beach 1979; Kriger 1992; Lan 1985; Bourdillon 1987; Machingura 2002). South Africans remember the names of Nxele, Nongqawuse and other resisting prophets (Peires 1982, Chapter 5; Peires 1989). In southern Tanzania, healers played a role in the great Maji Maji uprising.

In a colonial world where white conquest led to health crises and where healing prophets responded to those crises, the European colonizers saw healers as potentially dangerous opponents and tried to find ways to bring them under control and suppress their activities. In the British colonies, governments tried to control healers through the adoption and selective enforcement of anti-witchcraft ordinances (Feierman 1999; Mesaki 1997; Chavunduka 1980). These defined almost all the activities of traditional healers as witchcraft. By attacking healers, the governments played a role in defining the characteristic profile of traditional healing throughout the region. Healers everywhere in southeast Africa knew that they faced the possibility of persecution, so they went underground and practiced defensive medicine. They already had a sense, going back to the precolonial period, that important knowledge ought to be secret, since they needed secrecy to preserve their monopolies in societies where oral transmission made it possible for knowledge to circulate easily. Now secrecy was shaped in a slightly different way, since it served the purpose of keeping healers below the line of vision of colonial authorities. The difficult relationship between government and healers described in this book in relation to the changing roles of FRELIMO and AMETRAMO, therefore, has deep historical roots and is deeply embedded in regional patterns of healing authority.

Other elements of the region's traditional healing emerged in their current form as a result of colonial-period pressures. All across the region, Africans were drawn into the colonial cash economy. The best-known and most obvious manifestation of this was in patterns of oscillating migrant labor in which men left their homes to work for white-owned enterprises, whether on plantations, in mines, in cities, or on settler farms. The region's colonial rulers established an elaborate system of rewards and constraints to keep Africans' agricultural incomes at home low and move male labor from place to place: forced labor (in the early period everywhere, and in Mozambique for longer periods), head taxes, hut taxes, poll taxes, official labor recruitment agencies (like the Witwatersrand Native Labour Association), differential agricultural prices (to manipulate the probability that Africans could pay taxes by working on their own farms), land seizures, the structuring of the transport net, and a whole range of other measures.

The productive system had a profound effect on the shape of local health care. In this low-wage, low-social-service economy, Africans could not count on government or employers to provide a safety net. For the large majority of the region's working population, there was no retirement insurance, no disability insurance, and no health insurance for families. This meant that local clusters of kin had no choice but to organize and pay for their own health care. And this led to the particular shape of the region's health care, in which health care choices are made within family-based networks, in which patients move back and forth between hospitals and traditional healers, and in which traditional healers, in their treatments, deal not only with individual patients but with clusters of kin.

All this happened at a time when missionary church institutions, which had come in with European rule, chose not to emphasize spiritual healing, although (as we have seen) they did believe that providing scientifically based medical assistance was a part of their spiritual mission. Africans who found Christianity appealing but who wished to have healing as an integral part of their religious life could find congregations that satisfied them in these terms only within the separatist churches. These began to emerge in South Africa and Malawi in the late nineteenth and early twentieth centuries and then spread through the region (Sundkler 1961, Chapter 2; Pachai 1969; see essays by van Dijk, Pfeiffer, and Luedke in this volume). The negotiations described in this book about the boundaries between church and hospital and healing emerge from the historical patterns set back then.

The capacity of colonial power to shape African healing did not reach a terminal point in the late colonial period. Even over the past thirty years, as we see in the chapters of this book, the region's peoples have shared traumatic and formative experiences. The greater part of the late twentieth century was taken up with a violent struggle over the fate of white rule. That struggle unfolded in South Africa, in Zimbabwe, in Mozambique, and elsewhere in the region. The people of Mozambique, for example, suffered terrible disruptions. They fought a guerrilla war against their Portuguese rulers, who left in 1974, but after that ordinary people were caught in the midst of an internal war between the Mozambican government and RENAMO—violent and destructive rebels who were sponsored first by white-governed Rhodesia (that is, Zimbabwe) and then by South Africa. According to some estimates, more than 5 percent of the population died during the civil war, nearly 30 percent were displaced internally, and nearly 12 percent sought refuge in other countries (Ramsay 2004, 138–139). Zimbabwe, too, suffered a civil war, in this case between African guerrilla forces and the army created by the white minority regime. South Africa, by contrast, did not experience this kind of continuous warfare, but people suffered nonetheless. The white National Party government imprisoned, tortured, or murdered many people who opposed the regime, and the period's violence spilled over into political actions that separated Africans in South Africa from one another.

Healing practices proved themselves valuable in this context, during and after the periods of greatest violence. I reflected on this, and on the value of healing boundaries, during a visit to a Sabbath service of Amanazaretha, not far from Durban, in South Africa, in 1994, just after the country had achieved majority rule. The Amanazaretha are followers of the late Isaiah Shembe. They sing hymns to uNkulunkulu ka Shembe (the God of Shembe), hymns that had come to the founder in his dreams (see Sundkler 1961; Muller 1999). The service, which took place on a hilltop, was attended by 6,000 or 7,000 people, who were densely seated on mats in the open air. I arrived at an hour when most of the participants had already assembled, and I was being led along by the congregation's equivalent of ushers. When I saw a gap in the crowd where I might sit, I stepped into the crowd, only to be pulled back by my hosts, who were aghast that I had breached the boundary of the *itembeli*, the "temple." Rather than go to the entry, I had stepped across a line of white stones on the ground that constituted the boundary. The whitewashed stones—a mere line one stone high that barely reached my ankles—counted as though they were the wall of a tall cathedral.

I was especially struck by the fact that in this part of South Africa, where (at that moment) violent crime, theft, and political assassination were rife, the congregation of Amanazaretha was a kind of sanctuary. The thousands of people who attended the service left their purses and bags in a complete jumble before they went in, without markers of ownership, trusting that in this domain of religion and healing, they and their possessions would be safe. Just as precolonial territorial shrines defined invisible boundaries of a community that were different from the politically bounded ones, so the whitewashed stones were defining a world of safety that was outside normal politics.

Within the larger southeast African region, the period of violence was followed by one in which people found themselves in desperate need of individual healing; they also needed to rebuild their communities. But the international political and economic environment has not been a nurturing one. The period of open violence was followed by a more insidious, less noisy kind of violence—the quiet violence of powerlessness and disease, of life at the margin without a safety net. In Mozambique, economic liberalization required that poor people leave behind economic practices that were not market driven, that the better off be permitted to accumulate, and that government expenditures on health and education be cut back. The result was that poor people had a desperately hard time meeting basic needs, inequalities became much sharper, and it became more difficult (more costly, in a sense) for people to help one another without compensation. This environment has shaped the healing landscape just as profoundly as the colonial labor system did by raising the level of economic pressure, especially on poor women. In this context, at a time when the spirit of global economic liberalization is entering the heart even of traditional healing, the balance between traditional healers and healing churches is changing drastically. The churches are expanding because they take something of the form of older voluntary healing associations and because they offer help without a price tag attached.

If, in the current period of ongoing emergency, violence and pain "unmake" the world (as Luedke argues, following Scarry), then healers in a socially grounded tradition are uniquely well placed for remaking it. When the years of the greatest violence ended in Mozambique and Zimbabwe, healers took on the job of performing ceremonies to reintegrate victims of civil war into their communities, thus removing from them the pollution of violence and making it possible for them to live in a productive way alongside their neighbors. The victims were made to cross a boundary, to come in from a domain of violence to one of peaceful productivity. The perpetrators of violence were at least as much in need of crossing this boundary as the victims (Nordstrom 1997; Reynolds 1996). Mozambicans recognized, once the period of violent retribution against them had come to an end, that perpetrators both posed a danger and also had a deep need for healing.

If we look back over the long history that began with colonial conquest and ended with the decolonization struggles, we can see that healing in this cultural region was shaped by all these exogenous events and processes—by the shape of colonial political rule, the colonial economy, and colonial religion; by the process of decolonization; and by economic forces in the postcolonial world. All of these left profound imprints on local healing patterns. But the sources of similarity in the region's healing practices are not just external or colonial—they come also from a reliance on the region's rich and ancient body of cultural resources. The peoples of southeast Africa are heirs to a common heritage of understandings about the body, about misfortune, about the efficacy of material objects, and about social interventions that touch the body. Historians know something about this shared heritage because they are able to see ways the therapeutic understandings are encoded in the region's languages. They are able also to demonstrate that these languages stem from common origins and are very similar to one another. A comparison might help illustrate the nature of the similarity. If we think of the extent to which speakers of Spanish and Italian, in Europe, understand one another (in terms of both language and culture) we have a sense of shared similarities within southeast Africa. People within the region's societies speak closely related languages of what Ehret has called the Mashariki branch of the Bantu languages (Ehret 2001; Schoenbrun 2001; Vansina 2001; Batibo 2001). Communities that spoke the various languages began to separate from an ancestral speech community only relatively recently in terms of the timing of linguistic separation—perhaps 3,000 years ago, perhaps less. In any event, people who speak these languages find it relatively easy to understand one another's languages and therapeutic practices.

One example of these linguistically based cultural commonalities is in the term *nganga* or its cognates. The word *nganga* (which some translate as "healer") is in use across all the regions where Bantu languages are spoken. The *nganga*'s role is one, almost everywhere, that combines "the manufacturing of charms, the preparation and administration of herbal medicines, divination/diagnosis, ritual healing, witch detection" (Schoffeleers 1994, 75; see also Vansina 1990, 298). In addition, in the past, the *nganga* figures dealt with issues that concerned health and reproduction at a collective or public level. *Banganga* took measures to ensure that the rains fell in the proper season and they dealt with threats to successful agriculture: they used accepted means to manage pests that threatened crops and improve soil fertility. In many societies, they commented on public affairs and opposed political leaders whose actions endangered health and fertility (Feierman 1995; Schoffeleers 1992). At a deeper level, the work of *banganga* all across the region combines social or ritual or religious interventions with ones that are also material—not as two separate realms (social and material) that have been merged but as a single seamless domain of *uganga*. I am not arguing here that southeast Africa is a healing region because all the *nganga* figures practice in the same way. To say this would be incorrect. Rather, there is a regional style in the healers' practices, a set of themes and variations, so that people who responded to similar colonial challenges were able to draw on similar repertoires of cultural resources. This makes the regional study of themes and variations, as in this book, all the more rewarding.

Another commonality that characterizes all of Bantu-speaking Africa, and not merely the southeastern region, is the importance of healing associations. Groups of people band together voluntarily for healing purposes; each individual seeks his or her way to health but does it as part of a structured group (Janzen 1992). Initiation into group membership comes through healing rituals, so there is no separation between the process of therapy and that of the incorporation of members. Within the group, people often treat one another as though they were family. In the precolonial Lemba association, for example, near the Atlantic coast, an initiate would have a Lemba mother and a Lemba father—not instead of their own parents, but as a supportive group in the context of this particular mode of affliction (Janzen 1982). Becoming a Lemba daughter did not preclude remaining a daughter in kinship relations outside the association.

In southeast Africa, associations that focus around regional shrines have played a major role. The shrines were historically important, and some survive today. They draw people from scattered places of origin and usually deal with both individual and collective misfortunes. Werbner (1977), Garbett (1977), Nthoi (1998), and many other anthropologists have written about their structures, and Terence Ranger (1967) has shown how important they were historically for political mobilization. One example of how this works is given by Schoffeleers (1992), who writes about Mbona. In the Shire Valley of Malawi, from the seventeenth century onward, the collective health of an entire subregion (including the fertility of the rains) depended at least in part on the politics of a shrine to Mbona, a rainmaker who was killed by his enemies, whose blood was said to have become a lake, and who then manifested himself to people through storms and through a medium at a shrine built in his name. The land within which Mbona had influence was larger than the domain of any one chief. Mbona's boundaries, in other words, took in the territories of a number of smaller polities. In that period (as in this one), the power to heal existed in a fruitfully dynamic relationship with the power to transcend locality. In fact, Mbona could not end misfortune in the land unless a number of local political authorities from different places collaborated to build the shrine house. And it was Mbona's medium who could (at times, not always) speak with authority about the problems of the region (Schoffeleers 1992). At regional shrines in southeast Africa honoring other figures, individual illnesses were treated, as were collective ones.

Mbona and the other healing shrines illustrate the way that in these regional traditions, healing institutions constituted community in ways that cut across the political boundaries of parochial units of government. The relationship between healing and the fluidity of boundaries is one that was right at the heart of the region's precolonial political processes.

The rich regional healing culture of southeast Africa and of the larger Bantu-speaking region can be illustrated by endless additional examples of shared healing culture. First, many people in the region, today as in the past, rely on a kind of rough rule of thumb by which they separate two basic kinds of illnesses. One set is attributed to human anger or aggression or some other human cause, and the other set is defined as illnesses that just happen by themselves, without human agency, that can be situated in a world of material objects. A second common element in the region's healing cultures, and across the rest of Bantu-speaking Africa, is the relationship between the experience of illness and the path toward a healer's calling. The patient who suffers and tries to cure herself (or himself) with the help of an *nganga* can later also emerge as an *nganga*, using the skills she acquired during her own illness for healing others. People also become healers, all across the region, if they are chosen by a spirit or if they are capable of identifying the presence of the spirits (or a spirit) in others. All these, and others, are common patterns among the societies of the Bantu-speaking region. They do not lead to an identity of practice but rather to a rich profusion of practices that shares certain common elements underlying their diversity.

The deep similarities in therapeutic practice come not only from a shared heritage of related Bantu languages but also from a dramatic history of the movement and intermingling of populations, most dramatically in the period after 1880, but also even earlier. The southeast African region's archaeological record shows that Bantu-speaking peoples have engaged in trade for a very long time, have moved from place to place, and have borrowed bits of material culture from one another (Hall 1987). In other words, while some commonalities in the region's healing styles derive (as we have seen) from a shared inheritance within the broader Bantu-speaking community, still others emerge from the interaction of peoples in later periods. For example, Zulu-speaking armies began heading north from South Africa in the 1820s as a result of a regional political crisis. They helped found conquest states in a number of localities all the way up southeast Africa, as far as Tanzania. Along the way, the migrant groups interacted with local people. Often men who originated in Zululand married local women in the countries that today are called Zimbabwe, Mozambique, Malawi, Zambia, and Tanzania. In the process, healing practices that originated in South Africa mingled with northern ones, leading to the emergence of hybrid forms (Friedson 1996, 191n7). We can see, then, that the boundary-crossing that is at the heart of today's therapeutic practice, as described in the essays of this book, has a history that goes back to many different periods before European conquest.

With the coming of the colonial labor system, as we have seen, movement across the region increased. Workers from Lesotho and Mozambique went in great numbers to the South African mines. So many workers traveled the thousand miles from Malawi to South Africa to work as mine clerks and in other jobs that Bridglal Pachai (1969) has written about a "Malawi Diaspora." Clements Kadalie, the leader of the huge Industrial and Commercial Workers' Union in South Africa in the 1920s, was from Malawi, and the union had a major impact in Lesotho, Swaziland, Botswana, Malawi, Mozambique, Zambia, Zimbabwe, and Namibia (to use their postcolonial names) (Bradford 1987, 306n67).

The result of all this movement is that people learned one another's healing practices, and this was especially easy in a region where people shared the heritage of Bantu languages within a single linguistic subregion and where they had already experienced centuries of interaction.

The argument to this point identifies several discrete social processes, each of which contributes to the characteristic style of southeast African healing. The exercise of colonial power has shaped the traditional healing professions so that they have, until recently, preferred to work in the shadows, outside public view (Chavunduka 1980; Mesaki 1997). The low-wage colonial economy led to the centrality of lay management of therapy, since patients' kin were the only ones who would pay for treatment. At a different level, that of shared historical culture, ancient inherited patterns, encoded and reflected in language, led to the characteristic definition of the *nganga*'s role, the development of regional shrines, and the definition of a kind of regional folk epistemology.

This picture, which separates out levels of causation is, of course, oversimplified. I am not now turning around and rejecting my own generalization that family management of therapy met colonial-period needs, but I am adding to it. It is true also that therapy management by kin has a deep history that goes back long before colonial conquest. And it is obvious that the *nganga*'s role is not a static and traditional one; it is reshaped every day, in practice.

And then of course there is the hugely important role of circulation—of practices adopted today (and in the past) because people have seen them in another place or heard about them or read about them or saw them on the television or borrowed them from visiting healers. There are elements taken from Islamic healing and from the world of heterodox Islamic spirit practices. There is writing as healing technology—the washed words of Islamic medicines and the written formulae of books by and for traditional healers. There is the borrowing of forms of bureaucratic organization for healers' associations. There is the addition of Ayurvedic medicines from South Asia (borrowed as long ago as the late nineteenth century) to make them a part of the African traditional healer's medicine bag (Flint 2001). There is the addition of hypodermic syringes and white coats to the material culture of traditional healing. And there is the borrowing of many other practices, images, techniques, bits of clothing, gestures, and ideas.

The processes are, of course, too complex to capture. But taken all together, they add up to an unbounded, infinitely creative body of traditional medicine that, despite its fluidity and protean sense of movement, nevertheless expresses a powerful sense of place.

Note

1.   In fairness, it must be said that Evans-Pritchard expressed doubts, in the same essay, that regularities equivalent to those in the natural sciences would ever be found in anthropology (1963, 26–27).

References Cited

Abdool Karim, S. S., T. T. Ziqubu-Page, and R. Arendse. 1994. "Bridging the Gap: Potential for a Health Care Partnership between African Traditional Healers and Biomedical Personnel in South Africa." *South African Medical Journal* 84 (12): B1–B16.

Agha, Sohail, Andrew S. Karlyn, and Dominique Meekers. 2001. "The Promotion of Condom Use in Non-Regular Sexual Partnerships in Urban Mozambique." *Health Policy and Planning* 16 (2): 144–151.

Agrawal, Arun. 1995. "Dismantling the Divide between Indigenous and Scientific Knowledge." *Development and Change* 26 (3): 413–439.

———. 2002. "Indigenous Knowledge and the Politics of Classification." *International Social Science Journal* 54 (173): 287–297.

AMETRAMO. 1998. *Associação da Medicina Tradicional de Moçambique (AMETRAMO): Estatuto.* Maputo: Mozambique.

Anderson, Warwick. 2001. "Excremental Colonialism: Public Health and the Poetics of Pollution." In *Contagion: Historical and Cultural Studies*, ed. Alison Bashford and Claire Hooker, 76–105. London: Routledge.

Andersson, Jens A. 2001. "Mobile Workers, Urban Employment and 'Rural' Identities: Rural-Urban Networks of Buhera Migrants, Zimbabwe." In *Mobile Africa: Changing Patterns of Movement in Africa and Beyond*, ed. M. de Bruijn, R. van Dijk, and D. Foeken. Leiden: Brill.

———. 2002. "Sorcery in the Era of 'Henry IV': Kinship, Mobility and Mortality in Buhera District, Zimbabwe." *Journal of the Royal Anthropological Institute* 8 (3): 425–449.

Andersson, Neil, and Shula Marks. 1989. "The State, Class and the Allocation of Health Resources in Southern Africa." *Social Science and Medicine* 28 (5): 515–530.

Antze, Paul, and Michael Lambek. 1996. "Introduction: Forecasting Memory." In *Tense Past: Cultural Essays in Trauma and Memory*, ed. Paul Antze and Michael Lambek, xi–xxxviii. New York: Routledge.

Appadurai, Arjun. 1996. *Modernity at Large: Cultural Dimensions of Globalization.* Minneapolis: University of Minnesota Press.

Ashforth, Adam. 2000. *Madumo: A Man Bewitched.* Chicago: University of Chicago Press.

———. 2001. "On Living in a World with Witches: Everyday Epistemology and Spiritual Insecurity in a Modern African City (Soweto)." In *Magical Interpretations, Material Realities: Modernity, Witchcraft, and the Occult in Postcolonial Africa*, ed. H. L. Moore and T. Sanders, 206–225. New York: Routledge.

———. 2002. "An Epidemic of Witchcraft? The Implications of AIDS for the Post-Apartheid State." *African Studies* 61 (1): 121.

Auslander, Mark. 1993. "'Open the Wombs!': The Symbolic Politics of Modern Ngoni Witchfinding." In *Modernity and Its Malcontents: Ritual and Power in Postcolonial Africa*, ed. Jean Comaroff and John Comaroff, 167–192. Chicago: University of Chicago Press.

Austen, Ralph. 1993. "The Moral Economy of Witchcraft: An Essay on Comparative History." In *Modernity and Its Malcontents: Ritual and Power in Postcolonial Africa,* ed. Jean Comaroff and John Comaroff, 89–110. Chicago: University of Chicago Press.

Azevedo, Mario J. 2002. *Tragedy and Triumph: Mozambique Refugees in Southern Africa, 1977–2001.* Portsmouth, N.H.: Heinemann.

Badstuebner, Jennifer. 2003. "'Drinking the Hot Blood of Humans': Witchcraft Confessions in a South African Pentecostal Church." *Anthropology and Humanism* 28 (1): 8–22.

Bannerman, Robert H., John Burton, and Ch'en Wen-Chieh. 1983. *Traditional Medicine and Health Care Coverage: A Reader for Health Administrators and Practitioners.* Geneva: World Health Organization.

Barad, Karen. 1999. "Agential Realism: Feminist Interventions in Understanding Scientific Practices." In *The Science Studies Reader,* ed M. Biagioli, 1–11. New York: Routledge.

Barbour, Rosaline S., and Guro Huby, eds. 1998. *Meddling with Mythology: AIDS and the Social Construction of Knowledge.* London and New York: Routledge.

Basch, L., N. Glick Schiller, and C. Blanc-Szanton, eds. 1994. *Nations Unbound: Transnational Projects, Postcolonial Predicaments and Deterritorialized Nation-States.* Reading: Gordon & Breach Publishers.

Bashford, Alison. 2003. *Imperial Hygiene: A Critical History of Colonialism, Nationalism, and Public Health.* London: Palgrave.

Bashkow, Ira. 2004. "A Neo-Boasian Conception of Cultural Boundaries." *American Anthropologist* 106 (3): 443–458.

Bassett, M. T., L. Bijlmakers, and D. M. Sanders. 1997. "Professionalism, Patient Satisfaction, and Quality of Health Care: Experience during Zimbabwe's Structural Adjustment Programme." *Social Science and Medicine* 45 (12): 1845–1852.

Bastian, Misty L. 2001. "Vulture Men, Campus Cultists and Teenaged Witches: Modern Magics in Nigerian Popular Media." In *Magical Interpretations, Material Realities,* ed. H. L. Moore and T. Sanders, 71–96. New York: Routledge.

Bates, Don. 1995. "Scholarly Ways of Knowing: An Introduction." In *Knowledge and the Scholarly Medical Traditions,* ed. D. Bates, 1–22. Cambridge: Cambridge University Press.

Batibo, H. M. 2001. "Comment on Ehret, 'Bantu Expansions.'" *The International Journal of African Historical Studies* 34 (1): 68–70.

Bayart, Jean-François. 1993. *The State in Africa: The Politics of the Belly.* London and New York: Longman.

Beach, David. 1979. "Chimurenga: The Shona Rising of 1896–97." *Journal of African History* 20 (3): 395–420.

Beattie, John. 1963. "Sorcery in Bunyoro." In *Witchcraft and Sorcery in East Africa,* ed. J. Middleton and E. H. Winter, 27–55. London: Routledge & Kegan Paul.

Behrend, H., and U. Luig, eds. 1999. *Spirit Possession, Modernity & Power in Africa.* Oxford: James Currey.

Benjamin, Walter. 1968. *Illuminations: Essays and Reflections.* New York: Shocken Books.

Beyer, Peter. 1994. *Religion and Globalization.* London: Sage Publications.

———. 2001. *Religion in the Process of Globalization.* Hamburg: Ergon Verlag.

Bhabha, Homi. 1994. *The Location of Culture.* London and New York: Routledge.

Bierlich, Bernhard. 1999. "Sacrifice, Plants, and Western Pharmaceuticals: Money and Health Care in Northern Ghana." *Medical Anthropology Quarterly* 13 (3): 316–337.

Binsbergen, Wim van. 1995. "Four-Tablet Divination as Trans-Regional Medical Tech-
    nology in Southern Africa." *Journal of Religion in Africa* 25 (2): 114–140.
Bledsoe, Caroline. 1980. *Women and Marriage in Kpelle Society.* Stanford, Calif.: Stanford
    University Press.
Boddy, Janice. 1989. *Wombs and Alien Spirits: Women, Men, and the Zār Cult in Northern
    Sudan.* Madison: University of Wisconsin Press.
———. 1994. "Spirit Possession Revisited: Beyond Instrumentality." *Annual Review of
    Anthropology* 23: 407–434.
Bongmba, Elias K. 1998. "Toward a Hermeneutic of Wimbum Tfu." *African Studies Re-
    view* 41 (3): 165–191.
Boraine, Alex, and Janet Levy, eds. 1995. *The Healing of a Nation?* Cape Town, South
    Africa: Justice in Transition.
Boraine, Alex, Janet Levy, and Ronel Scheffer, eds. 1994. *Dealing with the Past: Truth and
    Reconciliation in South Africa.* Cape Town, South Africa: Institute for Democ-
    racy in South Africa.
Boswall, Karen. 1999. *From the Ashes.* Documentary film. Johannesburg, South Africa:
    South African Broadcasting Corporation.
Bourdillon, Michael. 1982/1998. *The Shona Peoples.* Gweru: Mambo Press.
———. 1987. "Guns and Rain: Taking Structural Analysis Too Far?" *Africa* 57 (2): 263–274.
———. 1991. *The Shona Peoples.* 3rd ed. Gweru, Zimbabwe: Mambo Press.
Bradford, Helen. 1987. *A Taste of Freedom: The ICU in Rural South Africa, 1924–1930.*
    New Haven, Conn., and London: Yale University Press.
Breslau, Joshua. 2000. "Globalizing Disaster Trauma: Psychiatry, Science, and Culture af-
    ter the Kobe Earthquake." *Ethos* 28 (2): 174–197.
Brodwin, Paul. 1996. *Medicine and Morality in Haiti: The Contest for Healing Power.*
    Cambridge and New York: Cambridge University Press.
Brouwer, Jan. 1998. "On Indigenous Knowledge and Development." *Current Anthro-
    pology* 39 (3): 351.
Brown, Karen McCarthy. 1989. "Afro-Caribbean Spirituality: A Haitian Case Study." In
    Healing and Restoring: Health and Medicine in the World's Religious Traditions,
    ed. L. E. Sullivan, 255–285. New York: Macmillan Publishing Company.
Bulhan, Hussein. 1993. "Imperialism in Studies of the Psyche: A Critique of African Psy-
    chological Research." In *Psychology and Oppression: Critiques and Proposals,* ed.
    Lionel Nicholas, 1–34. Johannesburg: Skotaville Publishers.
Burke, Charlanne. 2000. "They Cut Segametsi into Parts: Ritual Murder, Youth, and
    the Politics of Knowledge in Botswana." *Anthropological Quarterly* 73 (4): 204–
    214.
Butchart, Alex. 1998. *The Anatomy of Power: European Constructions of the African Body.*
    Pretoria: UNISA Press.
Callon, Michel. 1999. "Some Elements of a Sociology of Translation: Domestication of
    the Scallops and the Fisherman of St. Brieuc Bay." In *The Science Studies Reader,*
    ed. Mario Biagioli, 67–83. New York: Routledge.
Castanheira, Narciso. 1979. "Curandeiros Espiritistas: Desmascarar a Mentira." *Tempo*
    474 (11 November).
Chabal, Patrick, and Pascal Daloz. 1999. *Africa Works: Disorder as Political Instrument.*
    Bloomington: Indiana University Press.
Chakanza, J. C. 1985. *Provisional Annotated Chronological List of Witch-finding Move-
    ments in Malawi, 1850–1980.* Zomba, Malawi: Department of Religious Studies,
    Chancellor College.

Chalmers, Beverley. 1996. "Western and African Conceptualizations of Health." *Psychology and Health* 12 (1): 1–10.

Chapman, Rachel. In press. "Endangering Safe Motherhood in Mozambique: Prenatal Care as Reproductive Risk." *Social Science & Medicine.*

Chapman, Rachel, Paulino Davissone, Francisco Machobo, and James Pfeiffer. 1999. "Community Leadership and Health: A Rapid Ethnographic Study of Three Zones in Manica Province." Report prepared for the Mozambique Ministry of Health and Health Alliance International, Chimoio, Mozambique.

Chavunduka, G. L. 1978. *Traditional Healers and the Shona Patient.* Gwelo: Mambo Press.

———. 1980. "Witchcraft and the Law in Zimbabwe." *Zambezia* 8 (2): 129–147.

———. 1986. "The Organisation of Traditional Medicine in Zimbabwe." In *The Professionalisation of African Medicine,* ed. Murray Last and G. L. Chavunduka, 29–49. Manchester: Manchester University Press.

———. 1994. *Traditional Medicine in Modern Zimbabwe.* Harare, Zimbabwe: University of Zimbabwe Publications.

———. 1998. *The Professionalization of Traditional Medicine in Zimbabwe.* Harare, Zimbabwe: University of Zimbabwe Publications.

Chavunduka, Gordon L., and Murray Last. 1986. "African Medical Professions Today." In *The Professionalisation of African Medicine,* ed. M. Last and G. L. Chavunduka, 259–269. Manchester: International African Institute.

Clammer, John. 2002. "Beyond the Cognitive Paradigm: Majority Knowledges and Local Discourses in a Non-Western Society." In *Participating in Development: Approaches to Indigenous Knowledge,* ed. P. Sillitoe, A. Bicker, and J. Pottier, 43–63. London: Routledge.

Clark, Steve. 1999. *Travel Writing & Empire: Postcolonial Theory in Transit.* London and New York: Zed Books.

Cliff, Julie. 1991. "The War on Women in Mozambique: Health Consequences of South African Destabilization, Economic Crisis, and Structural Adjustment." In *Women and Health in Africa,* ed. Meredeth Turshen, 15–34. Trenton, N.J.: Africa World Press.

Cliff, Julie, and Abdul Razak Noormahomed. 1987. *The Impact on Health in Mozambique of South African Destabilization.* Maputo, Mozambique: Ministry of Health.

———. 1988. "Health as a Target: South Africa's Destabilization of Mozambique." *Social Science and Medicine* 27 (7): 717–722.

———. 1993. "The Impact of War on Children's Health in Mozambique." *Social Science and Medicine* 36 (7): 843–848.

Cliff, Julie, and Gill Walt. 1986. "The Dynamics of Health Policies in Mozambique 1975–85." *Health Policy and Planning* 1 (2): 148–157.

Cocks, Michelle, and Anthony Dold. 2000. "The Role of 'African Chemists' in the Health Care System of the Eastern Cape Province of South Africa." *Social Science and Medicine* 51 (10): 1505–1515.

Coleman, Simon. 2000. *The Globalization of Charismatic Christianity: Spreading the Gospel of Prosperity.* Cambridge: Cambridge University Press.

Colvin, Christopher. 2001a. "The Angel of Memory: 'Working Through' the History of the New South Africa." In *Between the Psyche and the Polis: Refiguring History in Literature and Theory,* ed. Michael Rossington and Anne Whitehead, 157–173. Aldershot: Ashgate Press.

———. 2001b. *"We Are Still Struggling": Storytelling, Reparations and Reconciliation after the TRC.* Johannesburg: Centre for the Study of Violence and Reconciliation.

———. 2004. "Performing the Signs of Injury: Critical Perspectives on Traumatic Storytelling after Apartheid." Ph.D. diss., University of Virginia.

Comaroff, Jean. 1985. *Body of Power, Spirit of Resistance: The Culture and History of a South African People.* Chicago: The University of Chicago Press.

Comaroff, Jean, and John L. Comaroff. 1991. *Of Revelation and Revolution.* Vol. 1, *Christianity, Colonialism, and Consciousness in South Africa.* Chicago: University of Chicago Press.

———. 1993. "Introduction." In *Modernity and Its Malcontents: Ritual and Power in Postcolonial Africa,* ed. Jean Comaroff and John Comaroff, xi–xxxvii. Chicago: University of Chicago Press.

———. 1997. *Of Revelation and Revolution.* Vol. 2, *The Dialectics of Modernity on a South African Frontier.* Chicago: University of Chicago Press.

———. 1999. "Occult Economies and the Violence of Abstraction: Notes from the South African Postcolony." *American Ethnologist* 26 (2): 279–303.

Comaroff, Jean, and John L. Comaroff, eds. 1993. *Modernity and Its Malcontents: Ritual and Power in Postcolonial Africa.* Chicago: University of Chicago Press.

Corten, Andre, and Ruth Marshall-Fratani, eds. 2001. *Between Babel and Pentecost: Transnational Pentecostalism in Africa and Latin America.* Bloomington: Indiana University Press.

Cox, Harvey. 1995. *Fire from Heaven: The Rise of Pentecostal Spirituality and the Reshaping of Religion in the Twenty-first Century.* Reading, Mass.: Addison-Wesley Publishing.

Crawford, J. R. 1967. *Witchcraft and Sorcery in Rhodesia.* London: International African Institute.

Daneel, Marthinus. 1970. *Zionism and Faith-Healing in Rhodesia.* The Hague: Mouton & Co.

———. 1988. *Old and New in Southern Shona Independent Churches.* Vol. 3, *Leadership and Fission Dynamics.* Gweru, Zimbabwe: Mambo Press.

———. 1992. "Exorcism as a Means of Combating Wizardry: Liberation or Enslavement." In *Empirical Studies of African Independent/Indigenous Churches,* ed. G. C. Oosthuizen and I. Hexham, 195–238. Lewiston, N.Y.: The Edwin Mellen Press.

Danfulani, Umar Habila Dadem. 1999. "Exorcising Witchcraft: The Return of the Gods in the New Religious Movements on the Jos Plateau and the Benue Regions of Nigeria." *African Affairs* 98 (391): 167–193.

Das, Veena, Arthur Kleinman, Mamphele Ramphele, and Pamela Reynolds, eds. 2000. *Violence and Subjectivity.* Berkeley: University of California Press.

Dauskardt, Rolf. 1991. "'Urban Herbalism': The Restructuring of Informal Survival in Johannesburg." In *South Africa's Informal Economy,* ed. E. Preston-Whyte and C. Rogerson, 87–100. Cape Town, South Africa: Oxford University Press.

Davis, Christopher O. 2000. *Death in Abeyance: Illness and Therapy among Tabwa of Central Africa.* Edinburgh: Edinburgh University Press for the International African Institute.

Davis, Wade. 1988. *Passage of Darkness: The Ethnobiology of the Haitian Zombie.* Chapel Hill: University of North Carolina Press.

Davis-Roberts, Christopher. 1992. "Kutambuwa Ugonjuwa: Concepts of Illness and

Transformation among the Tabwa of Zaire." In *The Social Basis of Health and Healing in Africa*, ed. S. Feierman and J. M. Janzen, 376–392. Berkeley: University of California Press.

Desjarlais, Robert, and Arthur Kleinman. 1994. "Violence and Demoralization in the New World Disorder." *Anthropology Today* 10 (5): 9–12.

Devisch, René. 1993. *Weaving the Threads of Life: The Khita Gyn-eco-logical Healing Cult among the Yaka*. Chicago: University of Chicago Press.

——. 1996. "'Pillaging Jesus': Healing Churches and the Villagisation of Kinshasa." *Africa* 66 (4): 555–585.

Dijk, Rijk van. 1992. "Young Puritan Preachers in Post-Independence Malawi." *Africa* 62 (2): 159–181.

——. 1995. "Fundamentalism and Its Moral Geography in Malawi: The Representation of the Diasporic and the Diabolical." *Critique of Anthropology* 15 (2): 171–191.

——. 1997. "From Camp to Encompassment: Discourses of Transsubjectivity in the Ghanaian Pentecostal Diaspora." *Journal of Religion in Africa* 27 (2): 135–159.

——. 1998. "Pentecostalism, Cultural Memory and the State: Contested Representations of Time in Postcolonial Malawi." In *Memory and the Postcolony: African Anthropology and the Critique of Power*, ed. Richard Werbner, 182–208. London: Zed Books.

——. 1999. "Pentecostalism, Gerontocratic Rule and Democratization in Malawi: The Changing Position of the Young in Political Culture." In *Religion, Globalization, and Political Culture in the Third World,* ed. J. Hayne. London: Macmillan.

——. 2001a. "Time and Transcultural Technologies of the Self in the Ghanaian Pentecostal Diaspora." In *Between Babel and Pentecost: Transnational Pentecostalism in Africa and Latin America*, ed. A. Corten and R. Marshall-Fratani. London and Bloomington: Hurst Publishers and Indiana University Press.

——. 2001b. "Witchcraft and Scepticism by Proxy: Pentecostalism and Laughter in Urban Malawi." In *Magical Interpretations, Material Realities: Modernity, Witchcraft and the Occult in Postcolonial Africa*, ed. H. L. Moore and T. Sanders, 97–117. New York: Routledge.

——. 2002a. "Localising Anxieties: Ghanaian and Malawian Immigrants, Rising Xenophobia, and Social Capital in Botswana." African Studies Centre Working Paper 49, Leiden, The Netherlands.

——. 2002b. "Religion, Reciprocity and Restructuring Family Responsibility in the Ghanaian Pentecostal Diaspora." In *The Transnational Family: New European Frontiers and Global Networks,* ed. D. F. Bryceson and V. Vuorela. Oxford: Berg.

——. 2003. "Localisation, Ghanaian Pentecostalism and the Stranger's Beauty in Botswana." *Africa* 73 (4): 560–583.

Dijk, Rijk van, Ria Reis, and Marja Spierenburg, eds. 2000a. *The Quest for Fruition through Ngoma: The Political Aspects of Healing in Southern Africa*. Athens: Ohio University Press; Oxford: James Currey.

——. 2000b. "Introduction: Beyond the Confinement of Affliction: A Discursive Field of Experience." In *The Quest for Fruition through Ngoma: The Political Aspects of Healing in Southern Africa,* ed. Rijk Van Dijk, Ria Reis, and Marja Spierenburg, 1–11. Oxford: James Currey.

Dillon-Malone, Clive. 1988. "Mutumwa Nchimi Healers and Wizardry Beliefs in Zambia." *Social Science and Medicine* 26 (11): 1159–1172.

Dube, D. 1989. "A Search for Abundant Life: Health, Healing and Wholeness in the Zionist Churches." In *Afro-Christian Religion and Healing in Southern Africa*, ed. G. C. Oosthuizen et al., 111–136. Lewiston, N.Y.: The Edwin Mellen Press.

Durkheim, Emile, and Marcel Mauss. 1903/1963. *Primitive Classification*. Translated, edited, with introduction by Rodney Needham. London: Cohen & West.

Eggan, Fred. 1954. "Social Anthropology and the Method of Controlled Comparison." *American Anthropologist* 56 (5): 743–763.

Ehret, Christopher. 2001. "Bantu Expansions: Re-envisioning a Central Problem of Early African History." *The International Journal of African Historical Studies* 34 (1): 5–41.

Eliade, Mircea. 1964. *Shamanism: Archaic Techniques of Ecstasy*. New York: Bollingen Foundation.

Ellen, Roy. 1998. "Response to Paul Sillitoe's 'The Development of Indigenous Knowledge: A New Applied Anthropology'." *Current Anthropology* 39 (2): 238–239.

———. 2002. "'Déja Vu, All Over Again,' Again: Reinvention and Progress in Applying Local Knowledge to Development." In *Participating in Development: Approaches to Indigenous Knowledge*, ed. P. Sillitoe, A. Bicker, and J. Pottier, 235–258. London: Routledge.

Ellis, Stephen. 1993. "Rumour and Power in Togo." *Africa* 63 (4): 462–475.

Englund, Harri. 1996. "Witchcraft, Modernity and the Person." *Critique of Anthropology* 16 (3): 257–279.

———. 2001. "The Quest for Missionaries. Transnationalism and Township Pentecostalism in Malawi." In *Between Babel and Pentecost: Transnational Pentecostalism in Africa and Latin America*, ed. A. Corten and R. Marshall-Fratani. London and Bloomington: Hurst Publishers and Indiana University Press.

Evans-Pritchard, Edward E. 1929/1967. "The Morphology and Function of Magic: A Comparative Study of Trobriand and Zande Rituals and Spells." In *Magic, Witchcraft, and Curing*, ed. J. Middleton, 1–22. Garden City, N.Y.: Natural History Press.

———. 1937. *Witchcraft, Oracles and Magic among the Azande*. Oxford: Clarendon Press.

———. 1937/1976. *Witchcraft, Oracles and Magic among the Azande*. Abridged ed. Oxford: Clarendon Press.

———. 1963. *The Comparative Method in Social Anthropology*. L. T. Hobhouse Memorial Trust Lecture, no. 33. London: The Athlone Press.

Farrell, Kirby. 1998. *Post-Traumatic Culture: Injury and Interpretation in the Nineties*. Baltimore, Md.: Johns Hopkins University Press.

Fauvet, P. 2000. "Mozambique: Growth with Poverty, a Difficult Transition from Prolonged War to Peace and Development." *Africa Recovery* 14 (3): 12–19.

Feierman, Steven. 1985. "Struggles for Control: The Social Roots of Health and Healing in Modern Africa." *African Studies Review* 28 (2/3): 73–147.

———. 1986. "Popular Control over the Institutions of Health: A Historical Study." In *The Professionalisation of African Medicine*, ed. M. Last and G. L. Chavunduka, 203–220. Manchester: International African Institute.

———. 1995. "Healing as Social Criticism in the Time of Colonial Conquest." *African Studies* (Johannesburg) 54 (1): 73–88.

———. 1999. "Colonizers, Scholars, and the Creation of Invisible Histories." In *Beyond the Cultural Turn: New Directions in the Study of Society and Culture*, ed. Victoria Bonnell and Lynn Hunt, 182–216. Berkeley: University of California Press.

Feierman, Steven, and John M. Janzen. 1992. "Introduction." In *The Social Basis of Health and Healing in Africa,* ed. S. Feierman and J. M. Janzen, 1–23. Berkeley: University of California Press.

Ferguson, James. 1999. *Expectations of Modernity: Myths and Meanings of Urban Life on the Zambian Copperbelt.* Berkeley: University of California Press.

———. 2002. "Of Mimicry and Membership: Africans and the 'New World Society.'" *Cultural Anthropology* 17 (4): 551–569.

Fernandez, James W. 1982. *Bwiti: An Ethnography of the Religious Imagination in Africa.* Princeton, N.J.: Princeton University Press.

Finnegan, William. 1992. *A Complicated War: The Harrowing of Mozambique.* Berkeley: University of California Press.

Flint, Karen. 2001. "Negotiating a Hybrid Medical Culture: African Healers in Southeastern Africa from the 1820s to the 1940s." Ph.D. diss., UCLA.

Flynn, Donna. 1997. "'We Are the Border': Identity, Exchange, and the State along the Benin-Nigeria Border." *American Ethnologist* 24 (2): 311–330.

Forster, Peter Glover. 1998. "Religion, Magic, Witchcraft, and AIDS in Malawi." *Anthropos* 93 (4–6): 537–544.

Fortes, Meyer. 1987. *Religion, Morality and the Person.* Cambridge: Cambridge University Press.

Friedson, Steven M. 1996. *Dancing Prophets: Musical Experience in Tumbuka Healing.* Chicago: University of Chicago Press.

Fry, Peter. 2000. "O Esirito Santo contra o Feitiço e os Espiritos Revoltados: 'Civilização' e 'Tradição' em Moçambique." *Mana* 6 (2): 65–95.

Garbett, Kingsley. 1977. "Disparate Regional Cults and a Unitary Field in Zimbabwe." In *Regional Cults,* ed. R. F. Werbner, 55–92. London: Academic Press.

Gaspar, Felisbela, and Armando Djedje. 1994. *Crenças e Práticas Tradicionais Relativas a Diarreia Infantil e as Doenças de Transmissão Sexual em Milange, Província da Zambézia: Relatório de Pesquisa e Comunicação.* Maputo: Gabineta de Estudos de Medicina Tradicional: Ministério da Saúde.

Geest, Sjaak van der. 1988. "The Articulation of Formal and Informal Medicine Distribution in South Cameroon." In *The Context of Medicines in Developing Countries,* ed. S. van der Geest and S. R. Whyte, 131–148. Dordrecht: Kluwer Academic Publishers.

———. 1997. "Is There a Role for Traditional Medicine in Basic Health Services in Africa? A Plea for a Community Perspective." *Tropical Medicine and International Health* 2 (9): 903–911.

Gelfand, Michael. 1962. *Shona Religion (with Special Reference to the Korekore).* Cape Town, South Africa: Juta.

———. 1964. *Witch Doctor: Traditional Medicine Man of Rhodesia.* London: Harvill Press.

Gelfand, Michael, S. Mavi, R. B. Drummond, and B. Ndemera. 1985. *The Traditional Medical Practitioner in Zimbabwe.* Gweru: Mambo Press.

Gennep, Arnold van. 1980/1960. *The Rites of Passage.* Translated by M. Vizedom and G. Caffee. London: Routledge & Kegan Paul.

Geschiere, Peter. 1997. *The Modernity of Witchcraft.* Charlottesville: University Press of Virginia.

———. 1998. "Globalization and the Power of Indeterminate Meaning: Witchcraft and Spirit Cults in Africa and East Asia." *Development and Change* 29 (4): 811–837.

———. 1999. "Globalization and the Power of Indeterminate Meaning: Witchcraft and Spirit Cults in Africa and East Asia." In *Globalization and Identity: Dialectics of*

Flow and Closure, ed. B. Meyer and P. Geschiere, 211–237. Oxford: Blackwell Publishers.

Geschiere, Peter, and Birgit Meyer. 1999. "Globalization and Identity: Dialectics of Flow and Closure." In *Globalization and Identity: Dialectics of Flow and Closure,* ed. B. Meyer and P. Geschiere, 1–15. Oxford: Blackwell Publishers.

Gieryn, Thomas F. 1983. "Boundary-Work and the Demarcation of Science from Non-Science." *American Sociological Review* 48 (6): 781–795.

Gifford, Paul. 1991. *The New Crusaders: Christianity and the New Right in Southern Africa.* London: Pluto Press.

———. 1994. "Ghana's Charismatic Churches." *Journal of Religion in Africa* 24 (3): 241–265.

———. 1998. *African Christianity: Its Public Role.* London: Hurst & Company.

Gifford, Paul, ed. 1995. *The Christian Churches and the Democratization of Africa.* Leiden: E. J. Brill.

Gluckman, Max. 1956. *Custom and Conflict in Africa.* Oxford: Basil Blackwell.

Good, Byron. 1994. *Medicine, Rationality, and Experience: An Anthropological Perspective.* Cambridge: Cambridge University Press.

Good, Charles M. 1987. *Ethnomedical Systems in Africa: Patterns of Traditional Medicine in Rural and Urban Kenya.* New York: Guilford Press.

Gray, Robert F. 1969. "The Shetani Cult among the Segeju of Tanzania." In *Spirit Mediumship and Society in Africa,* ed. J. Beattie and J. Middleton, 171–187. London: Routledge & Kegan Paul.

Green, Edward C. 1994. *AIDS and STDS in Africa: Bridging the Gap between Traditional Healing and Modern Medicine.* Boulder, Colo.: Westview Press.

———. 1996. *Indigenous Healers and the African State: Policy Issues concerning African Indigenous Healers in Mozambique and Southern Africa.* New York: Pact Publications.

———. 1997. "Purity, Pollution and the Invisible Snake in Southern Africa." *Medical Anthropology* 17 (1): 83–100.

———. 1999. *Indigenous Theories of Contagious Disease.* Walnut Creek, Calif.: AltaMira Press.

Green, Edward C., Annemarie Jurg, and Armando Dgedge. 1993. "Sexually-Transmitted Diseases, AIDs and Traditional Healers in Mozambique." *Medical Anthropology* 15 (3): 261–281.

———. 1994. "The Snake in the Stomach: Child Diarrhea in Central Mozambique." *Medical Anthropology Quarterly* 8 (1): 4–24.

Green, Edward C., Josefa Marrato, and Manuel Wilsonne. 1995. *Ethnomedical Study of Diarrheal Disease, AIDS/STDS and Mental Health in Nampula, Mozambique.* Maputo: Department of Traditional Medicine, Mozambique Ministry of Health.

Green, Maia. 1994. "Shaving Witchcraft in Ulanga." In *Witchcraft in Contemporary Tanzania,* ed. R. G. Abrahams, 23–45. Cambridge: African Studies Centre, University of Cambridge.

———. 1997. "Witchcraft Suppression Practices and Movements: Public Politics and the Logic of Purification." *Comparative Studies in Society and History* 39 (2): 319–345.

Greenwood, Bernard. 1992. "Cold or Spirits? Ambiguity and Syncretism in Moroccan Therapeutics." In *The Social Basis of Health and Healing in Africa,* ed. S. Feierman and J. M. Janzen, 285–314. Berkeley: University of California Press.

Griffin, Susan. 1978. *Women and Nature: The Roaring Inside Her.* New York: Harper and Row.

Guyer, Jane. 1996. "Traditions of Invention in Equatorial Africa." *African Studies Review* 39 (3): 1–28.

Guyer, Jane, and Eno Belinga. 1995. "Wealth in People as Wealth in Knowledge: Accumulation and Composition in Equatorial Africa." *Journal of African History* 36 (1): 91–120.

Hackett, R. I. J. 1998. "Charismatic/Pentecostal Appropriation of Media Technologies in Nigeria and Ghana." *Journal of Religion in Africa* 28 (3): 258–277.

Hacking, Ian. 1995. *Rewriting the Soul: Multiple Personality and the Sciences of Memory.* Princeton, N.J.: Princeton University Press.

———. 1996. "Memory Science, Memory Politics." In *Tense Past: Cultural Essays in Trauma and Memory,* ed. Paul Antze and Michael Lambek, 67–88. New York: Routledge.

Hall, Margaret. 1990. "The Mozambican National Resistance Movement (RENAMO): A Study in the Destruction of an African Country." *Africa* 60 (1): 39–68.

Hall, Martin. 1987. *The Changing Past: Farmers, Kings and Traders in Southern Africa, 200–1860.* Cape Town and Johannesburg: David Philip.

Hamber, Brandon. 1997. *The Burdens of Truth: An Evaluation of the Psychological Support Services and Initiatives Undertaken by the South African Truth and Reconciliation Commission.* Johannesburg: Centre for the Study of Violence and Reconciliation.

Hanlon, Joseph. 1991. *Mozambique: Who Calls the Shots?* London: James Currey.

———. 1996. *Peace without Profit: How the IMF Blocks Rebuilding in Mozambique.* Oxford: James Currey.

Hannerz, Ulf. 1987. "The World in Creolisation." *Africa* 57 (4): 546–559.

———. 1997. "Borders." *International Social Science Journal* 49 (4): 537–548.

Haraway, Donna. 1989. *Primate Visions: Gender, Race, and the Nature in the World of Modern Science.* New York: Routledge.

———. 1991. *Simians, Cyborgs, and Women: The Reinvention of Nature.* London: Free Association.

Haar, Gerrie ter, and Stephen Ellis. 1988. "Spirit Possession and Healing in Modern Zambia: An Analysis of Letters to Archbishop Milingo." *African Affairs* 87 (347): 185–206.

Harries, Patrick. 2001. "Missionaries, Marxists and Magic: Power and the Politics of Literacy in South-East Africa." *Journal of Southern African Studies* 27 (3): 405–427.

Heidegger, Martin. 1971. *Building, Dwelling, Thinking: Poetry, Language, Thought.* Translated by Albert Hofstadter. New York: Harper Colophon Books.

Herman, Judith. 1992. *Trauma and Recovery: From Domestic Abuse to Political Terror.* New York: Basic Books.

Hexham, I., and K. Poewe. 1997. *New Religions as Global Cultures: Making the Human Sacred.* Boulder, Colo.: Westview Press.

Hofmeyr, Isabel. 1991. "Jonah and the Swallowing Monster: Orality and Literacy on a Berlin Mission Station in the Transvaal." *Journal of Southern African Studies* 17 (4): 633–653.

Hongoro, C., and S. Chandiwana. 1994. *Effects of User Fees on Health Care in Zimbabwe.* Harare, Zimbabwe: Blair Research Institute.

Honwana, Alcinda Manuel. 1999. "The Collective Body: Challenging Western Concepts of Trauma and Healing." *Track Two* 1: 30–35.

———. 2002. *Espíritos Vivos, Tradições Modernas: Possessão de Espíritos e Reintegração Social Pós-Guerra no Sul de Moçambique.* Maputo: Promédia.

Howes, Michael, and Robert Chambers. 1980. "Indigenous Technical Knowledge: Analysis, Implications and Issues." In *Indigenous Knowledge Systems and Development,* ed. D. Brokensha, D. M. Warren, and O. Werner, 323–334. Lanham, Md.: University Press of America.

Humphrey, Caroline, and Urgunge Onon. 1996. *Shamans and Elders: Experience, Knowledge and Power among the Daur Mongols.* Oxford: Clarendon Press.

Hunt, Nancy Rose. 1999. *A Colonial Lexicon: Of Birth Ritual, Medicalization, and Mobility in the Congo.* Durham, N.C.: Duke University Press.

Iliffe, John. 1979. *A Modern History of Tanganyika.* Cambridge: Cambridge University Press.

———. 1990. *Famine in Zimbabwe, 1890–1960.* Gweru: Mambo Press.

———. 1998. *East African Doctors: A History of the Modern Profession.* Cambridge: Cambridge University Press.

INE (Instituto Nacional de Estatistica). 1998. *Inquerito Nacional aos Agregados Familiares Sobre Condicoes de Vida –1996–1997* [*National Family Survey on Living Conditions*]. Maputo: Government of Mozambique.

———. 1999. *II Recenseamento Geral da População e Habitação, 1997: Provincia de Manica* [*Second General Census: Manica Province*]. Maputo: Government of Mozambique.

Ingstad, Benedicte. 1989. "Healer, Witch, Prophet, or Modern Health Worker? The Changing Role of Ngaka ya Setswana." In *Culture, Experience, and Pluralism: Essays on African Ideas of Illness and Healing,* ed. A. Jacobson-Widding and D. Westerlund, 247–276. Uppsala: Academiae Upsaliensis.

———. 1990. "The Cultural Construction of AIDS and Its Consequences for Prevention in Botswana." *Medical Anthropology Quarterly* 4 (1): 28–40.

Isaacman, Allen, and Barbara Isaacman. 1976. *The Tradition of Resistance in Mozambique: Anti-Colonial Activity in the Zambesi Valley, 1850–1921.* Berkeley and Los Angeles: University of California Press.

———. 2004. *Slavery and Beyond: The Making of Men and Chikunda Ethnic Identities in the Unstable World of South-Central Africa, 1750–1920.* Portsmouth, N.H.: Heinemann.

Jansen, P. C. M., and Orlando Mendes. 1983–1984. *Plantas Medicinais: Seu Uso Tradicional em Moçambique.* Maputo: Gabineta de Estudos de Medicina Tradicional: Ministério da Saúde: República Popular de Moçambique.

Janzen, John M. 1978. *The Quest for Therapy: Medical Pluralism in Lower Zaire.* Berkeley: University of California Press.

———. 1982. *Lemba, 1650–1930: A Drum of Affliction in Africa and the New World.* New York and London: Garland Publishing.

———. 1985. "Changing Concepts of African Therapeutics: An Historical Perspective." In *African Healing Strategies,* ed. B. M. du Toit and I. H. Abdalla, 61–81. Owerri [Nigeria] and New York: Trado-Medic Books.

———. 1989. "Health, Religion, and Medicine in Central and Southern African Traditions." In *Healing and Restoring: Health and Medicine in the World's Religious Traditions,* ed. L. E. Sullivan, 225–254. New York: Macmillan Publishing Company.

———. 1992. *Ngoma: Discourses of Healing in Central and Southern Africa.* Berkeley: University of California Press.

———. 2001. "Afterword." In *The Quest for Fruition through Ngoma: Political Aspects of Healing in Southern Africa,* ed. Rijk van Dijk, Ria Reis, and Marja Spierenburg, 155–168. Cape Town, South Africa: David Philips.

Jefferis, K. 1998. "Botswana and Diamond-dependent Development." In *Botswana: Poli-*

tics and Society, ed. W. A. Edge and M. H. Lekorwe. Pretoria: J. L. van Schaik Publishers.

Jefferis K., and T. F. Kelly. 1999. "Botswana: Poverty amid Plenty." *Oxford Development Studies* 27 (2): 211–232.

Jenkins, Philip. 2002. *The Next Christendom: The Coming of Global Christianity.* Oxford: Oxford University Press.

Jilek-Aall, Louise. 1979. *Call Mama Doctor: African Notes of a Young Woman Doctor.* Saanichton, B.C., and Seattle, Wash.: Hancock House Publishers.

Kapferer, Bruce. 1997. *The Feast of the Sorcerer: Practices of Consciousness and Power.* Chicago: University of Chicago Press.

Karlyn, Andrew S. 2001. "The Impact of a Targeted Radio Campaign to Prevent STIs and HIV/AIDS in Mozambique." *AIDS Education and Prevention* 13 (5): 438–451.

Kearney, Michael. 1991. "Borders and Boundaries of State and Self at the End of Empire." *Journal of Historical Sociology* 4 (1): 52–74.

Keller, Evelyn Fox. 1985. *Reflections on Gender and Science.* New Haven, Conn.: Yale University Press.

———. 1992. *Secrets of Life/Secrets of Death: Essays on Language, Gender and Science.* New York and London: Routledge.

Kiernan, J. P. 1976a. "Prophet and Preacher: An Essential Partnership in the Work of Zion." *Man* 11 (3): 356–366.

———. 1976b. "The Work of Zion: An Analysis of an African Zionist Ritual." *Africa* 46 (4): 340–355.

———. 1977. "Poor and Puritan: An Attempt to View Zionism as a Collective Response to Urban Poverty." *African Studies* 36 (1): 31–41.

———. 1990. *The Production and Management of Therapeutic Power in Zionist Churches within a Zulu City.* Lewiston, N.Y.: The Edwin Mellen Press.

Knipe, David. 1989. "Hinduism and the Tradition of Ayurveda." In *Healing and Restoring: Health and Medicine in the World's Religious Traditions*, ed. L. E. Sullivan, 89–109. New York: Macmillan Publishing Company.

Kohnert, Dirk. 1996. "Magic and Witchcraft: Implications for Democratization and Poverty-Alleviating Aid in Africa." *World Development* 24: 1347–1355.

Kolk, Bessel A. van der, Alexander C. MacFarlane, and Lars Weisaeth, eds. 1995. *Traumatic Stress: The Effects of Overwhelming Experience on Mind, Body, and Society.* New York: Guilford Press.

Kriger, Norma. 1992. *Zimbabwe's Guerrilla War: Peasant Voices.* Cambridge: Cambridge University Press.

Krog, Antjie. 1998. *Country of My Skull.* Johannesburg: Random House.

Lalu, Premesh, and Brent Harris. 1996. "Journeys from the Horizons of History: Text, Trial and Tales in the Construction of Narratives of Pain." *Current Writing* 8 (2): 24–38.

Lambek, Michael. 1993. *Knowledge and Practice in Mayotte: Local Discourses of Islam, Sorcery, and Spirit Possession.* Toronto: University of Toronto Press.

Lan, David. 1985. *Guns and Rain: Guerillas and Spirit Mediums in Zimbabwe.* London: James Currey.

Langford, Jean M. 2002. *Fluent Bodies: Ayurvedic Remedies for Postcolonial Imbalance.* Durham, N.C.: Duke University Press.

Last, Murray. 1992. "The Importance of Knowing about Not Knowing: Observations from Hausaland." In *The Social Basis of Health and Healing in Africa*, ed. S. Feierman and J. M. Janzen, 393–406. Berkeley: University of California Press.

Last, Murray, and G. L. Chavunduka, eds. 1986. *The Professionalisation of African Medicine.* Manchester: Manchester University Press.

Latour, Bruno. 1988. *The Pasteurization of France.* Translated by Alan Sheridan and John Law. Cambridge, Mass.: Harvard University Press.

———. 1999. *Pandora's Hope: Essays on the Reality of Science Studies.* Cambridge, Mass.: Harvard University Press.

Leslie, Charles. 1976. "Introduction." In *Asian Medical Systems: A Comparative Study,* ed. C. Leslie, 1–12. Berkeley: University of California Press.

LeVine, Robert A. 1963. "Witchcraft and Sorcery in a Gusii Community." In *Witchcraft and Sorcery in East Africa,* ed. J. Middleton and E. H. Winter, 221–255. London: Routledge and Kegan Paul.

Lewis, Sharon. 1999. *An Adult's Guide to Childhood Trauma: Understanding Traumatised Children in South Africa.* Cape Town, South Africa: David Philip Publishers.

Leys, Ruth. 2000. *Trauma: A Genealogy.* Chicago: University of Chicago Press.

Liebenow, J. Gus. 1971. *Colonial Rule and Political Development in Tanzania: The Case of the Makonde.* Evanston, Ill.: Northwestern University Press.

Loewenson, Rand, and M. Chisvo. 1994. *Transforming Social Development: The Experience of Zimbabwe.* Harare, Zimbabwe: UNICEF.

Luig, Ute. 1999. "Constructing Local Worlds: Spirit Possession in the Gwembe Valley, Zambia." In *Spirit Possession, Modernity and Power in Africa,* ed. H. Behrend and U. Luig, 124–141. Madison: University of Wisconsin Press.

MacGaffey, Wyatt. 1983. *Modern Kongo Prophets: Religion in a Plural Society.* Bloomington: Indiana University Press.

MacGregor, Hayley. 2002. "Maintaining a Fine Balance: Negotiating Mental Distress in Khayelitsha, South Africa." Ph.D. diss., University of Cambridge.

Machingura, P. 2002. "Change." On *We Are Still Here.* Privately produced CD.

MacLeod, Roy, ed. 2000. *Colonialism and Science. Osiris,* vol. 15. Chicago: University of Chicago Press.

Mahlke, Reiner. 1995. "Aspects of Healing in Zionist Churches in South Africa." *Africana Marburgensia* 28 (1/2): 14–31.

Malkki, Liisa H. 1995. *Purity and Exile: Violence, Memory, and National Cosmology among Hutu Refugees in Tanzania.* Chicago: University of Chicago Press.

Manuh, T. 1998. "Ghanaians, Ghanaian Canadians, and Asantes: Citizenship and Identity among Migrants in Toronto." *Africa Today* 45 (3/4): 481–494.

Marshall, J. 1990. "Structural Adjustment and Social Policy in Mozambique." *Review of African Political Economy* 17 (48): 28–43.

Marwick, Max. 1950. "Another Modern Anti-Witchcraft Movement." *Africa* 20 (1): 100–112.

———. 1965. *Sorcery in Its Social Setting: A Study of the Northern Rhodesia Cewa.* Manchester: Manchester University Press.

Masquelier, Adeline. 2002. "Road Mythographies." *American Ethnologist* 29 (4): 829–856.

Maxwell, David. 1995. "Witches, Prophets and Avenging Spirits: The Second Christian Movement in North-East Zimbabwe." *Journal of Religion in Africa* 25: 309–339.

———. 1998. "'Delivered from the Spirit of Poverty?' Pentecostalism, Prosperity and Modernity in Zimbabwe." *Journal of Religion in Africa* 28 (3): 350–373.

———. 1999. "Historicizing Christian Independency: The Southern African Pentecostal Movement c. 1908–60." *Journal of African History* 40: 243–264.

Mbembe, Achille. 1992. "Provisional Notes on the Postcolony." *Africa* 62 (1): 3–37.

Meister, Robert. 1999. "After Evil: Moral Logics of National Recovery in the TRC Final

Report." Presented at the conference Commissioning the Past, University of Witwatersrand, Johannesburg, South Africa, June 11–14, 1999.

Meneses, M. Paula G. n.d. "'When there are no problems, we are healthy, no bad luck, nothing': Towards an Emancipatory Understanding of Health and Medicine." Centro de Estudos Sociais, Universidade de Coimbra. Available online at http://www.ces.fe.uc.pt/emancipa/research/en/saberes.html.

Merchant, Carolyn. 1990. *The Death of Nature: Women, Ecology, and the Scientific Revolution.* 2nd ed. San Francisco: Harper.

Merwe, Hugo van der, Polly DeWhirst, and Brandon Hamber. 1999. "Non-Governmental Organisations and the Truth and Reconciliation Commission: An Impact Assessment." *Politikon* 26 (1): 55–79.

Mesaki, Simeon. 1997. "The Colonial State and Witchcraft: Moral Crusade or Ethnocentric Phobia: The Case of British Colonialism in Tanganyika." *Tanzania Zamani* 3 (1): 50–71.

Meyer, Birgit. 1993. "'If you are a devil, you are a witch and if you are a witch, you are a devil': The Integration of 'Pagan' Ideas into the Conceptual Universe of Ewe Christians in Southeastern Ghana." In *Power and Prayer,* ed. Mart Bax and Adrianus Koster, 159–182. Amsterdam: VU University Press.

———. 1998. "'Make a Complete Break with the Past': Memory and Postcolonial Modernity in Ghanaian Pentecostal Discourse." In *Memory and the Postcolony: African Anthropology and the Critique of Power,* ed. Richard Werbner, 182–208. London: Zed Books.

Meyer, Birgit, and Peter Geschiere, eds. 1999. *Globalization and Identity: Dialectics of Flow and Closure.* Oxford: Blackwell Publishers.

Middleton, John, and E. H. Winter, eds. 1963. *Witchcraft and Sorcery in East Africa.* London: Routledge and Kegan Paul.

Ministry of Health, Mozambique. 1997. *Mozambique Demographic and Health Survey.* Maputo: Mozambique Ministry of Health and Macro International.

Ministry of Planning and Finance, Mozambique. 1998. *Understanding Poverty and Well-Being in Mozambique: The First National Assessment (1996–97).* Maputo: Government of Mozambique.

Minter, William. 1989. "The Mozambican National Resistance (RENAMO) as Described by Ex-Participants." *Development Dialogue* 1: 89–132.

Mitchell, Timothy. 1988. *Colonizing Egypt.* New York: Cambridge University Press.

Mogensen, Hanne Overgaard. 1997. "The Narrative of AIDS among the Tonga of Zambia." *Social Science and Medicine* 44 (4): 431–439.

Moore, Henrietta, and Todd Sanders, eds. 2001. *Magical Interpretations, Material Realities: Modernity, Witchcraft and the Occult in Postcolonial Africa.* London: Routledge.

Moore, Henrietta, and Megan Vaughan. 1994. *Cutting Down Trees: Gender, Nutrition, and Agricultural Change in the Northern Province of Zambia, 1890–1990.* Portsmouth, N.H.: Heinemann.

Morgan, Glenda. 1990. "Violence in Mozambique: Towards an Understanding of RENAMO." *The Journal of Modern African Studies* 28 (4): 603–619.

Mosha, A. C. 1998. "The Impact of Urbanisation on the Society, Economy and Environment of Botswana." In *Botswana: Politics and Society,* ed. W. A. Edge and M. H. Lekorwe. Pretoria: J. L. van Schaik Publishers.

Muller, Carol. 1999. *Rituals of Fertility and the Sacrifice of Desire: Nazarite Women's Performance in South Africa.* Chicago: University of Chicago Press.

Musambachime, Mwelwa C. 1988. "The Impact of Rumor: The Case of the Banyama (Vampire Men) Scare in Northern Rhodesia, 1930–1964." *The International Journal of African Historical Studies* 21 (2): 201–215.

Needham, Rodney. 1972. *Belief, Language, and Experience.* Oxford: Blackwell.

Ngubane, Harriet. 1992. "Clinical Practice and Organization of Indigenous Healers in South Africa." In *The Social Basis of Health and Healing in Africa,* ed. S. Feierman and J. M. Janzen, 366–375. Berkeley: University of California Press.

Nicholas, Lionel, ed. 1993. *Psychology and Oppression: Critiques and Proposals.* Johannesburg: Skotaville.

Nordstrom, Carolyn. 1997. *A Different Kind of War Story.* Philadelphia: University of Pennsylvania Press.

Nthoi, Leslie S. 1998. "Wosana Rite of Passage: Reflections on the Initiation of Wosana in the Cult of Mwali in Zimbabwe." In *Rites of Passage in Contemporary Africa: Interaction between Christian and African Traditional Religions,* ed. James L. Cox, 63–93. Cardiff, Wales: Cardiff Academic Press.

Nuttall, Mark. 1998. "Critical Reflections on Knowledge Gathering in the Arctic." In *Aboriginal Environmental Knowledge in the North,* ed. Louis-Jacques Dorais, Murielle Ida Nagy, and Ludger Müller-Wille, 21–35. Québec: Université Laval.

Nyamnjoh, Francis B. 2001. "Delusions of Development and the Enrichment of Witchcraft Discourses in Cameroon." In *Magical Interpretations, Material Realities: Modernity, Witchcraft and the Occult in Postcolonial Africa,* ed. H. L. Moore and T. Sanders, 28–49. New York: Routledge.

———. 2002. "Local Attitudes towards Citizenship and Foreigners in Botswana: An Appraisal of Recent Press Stories." *Journal of Southern African Studies* 28 (4): 755–775.

Obbo, Christine. 1996. "Healing, Cultural Fundamentalism and Syncretism in Buganda." *Africa* 66 (2): 183–201.

Oosthuizen, Gerhardus C. 1989. "Indigenous Healing within the Context of the African Independent Churches." In *Afro-Christian Religion and Healing in Southern Africa,* ed. G. C. Oosthuizen et al., 73–90. Lewiston, N.Y.: The Edwin Mellen Press.

———. 1992. *The Healer-Prophet in Afro-Christian Churches.* Leiden: E. J. Brill.

Otlhogile, B. 1994. *A History of the Higher Courts of Botswana, 1912–1990.* Gaborone, Botswana: Mmegi Publishing House.

Oucho, J. O. 2000. "Skilled Immigrants in Botswana: A Stable but Temporary Workforce." *Africa Insight* 30 (2): 56–65.

Pachai, Bridglal. 1969. *The Malawi Diaspora and Elements of Clements Kadalie.* The Central Africa Historical Association, Local Series Pamphlet 24. Salisbury, Southern Rhodesia: Central Africa Historical Association.

Pakleppa, Richard. 1999. *I Have Seen (Nda Mona).* Film. Johannesburg, South Africa: South African Broadcasting Corporation.

Parry-Jones, Brenda, and William L. L. Parry-Jones. 1994. "Post-Traumatic Stress Disorder: Supportive Evidence from an Eighteenth Century Natural Disaster." *Psychological Medicine* 24 (1): 15–27.

Pearce, Tola. 1986. "Professional Interests and the Creation of Medical Knowledge in Nigeria." In *The Professionalisation of African Medicine,* ed. M. Last and G. L. Chavunduka, 237–258. Manchester: International African Institute.

Peil, M. 1995. "Ghanaians Abroad." *African Affairs* 94 (376): 345–367.

Peires, Jeffrey. 1982. *The House of Phalo: A History of the Xhosa People in the Days of Their Independence.* Berkeley: University of California Press.

———. 1989. *The Dead Will Arise: Nongqawuse and the Great Xhosa Cattle-Killing Movement of 1856–7*. Johannesburg: Ravan Press.

Peletz, Michael G. 1993. "Knowledge, Power, and Personal Misfortune in a Malay Context." In *Understanding Witchcraft and Sorcery in Southeast Asia*, ed. C. W. Watson and R. F. Ellen, 149–177. Honolulu: University of Hawaii Press.

Pels, Peter. 1999. *A Politics of Presence: Contacts between Missionaries and Waluguru in Late Colonial Tanganyika*. Amsterdam: Harwood Academic.

Pfeiffer, James. 2002. "African Independent Churches in Mozambique: Healing the Afflictions of Inequality." *Medical Anthropology Quarterly* 16 (2): 176–199.

Pfeiffer, James, S. Gloyd, and L. Li. 2001. "Intrahousehold Resource Allocation and Child Growth in Central Mozambique: An Ethnographic Case-Control Study." *Social Science & Medicine* 53 (1): 83–97.

Pigg, Stacy Leigh. 1996. "The Credible and the Credulous: The Question of 'Villagers' Beliefs' in Nepal." *Cultural Anthropology* 11 (2): 160–201.

Pityana, N. Barney. 1995. "Outlook on the Month." *South African Outlook* 125 (6): 50–51.

Plotkin, Mark J. 1993. *Tales of a Shaman's Apprentice: An Ethnobotanist Searches for New Medicines in the Amazon Rain Forest*. New York: Viking.

Poewe, Karla, ed. 1994. *Charismatic Christianity as a Global Culture*. Columbia: University of South Carolina Press.

Portes, A. 1998. *Globalization from Below: The Rise of Transnational Communities*. Oxford: Transnational Communities Programme.

Posey, Darrell. 1990. "Intellectual Property Rights and Just Compensation of Indigenous Knowledge." *Anthropology Today* 6 (4): 13–16.

Prakash, Gyan. 1999. *Another Reason: Science and the Imagination of Modern India*. Princeton, N.J.: Princeton University Press.

Pratt, Mary Louise. 1992. *Imperial Eyes: Travel Writing and Transculturation*. London and New York: Routledge.

Prince, Ruth, and P. Wenzel Geissler. 2001. "Becoming 'One Who Treats': A Case Study of a Luo Healer and Her Grandson in Western Kenya." *Anthropology and Education Quarterly* 32 (4): 447–471.

Prins, Gwyn. 1992. "A Modern History of Lozi Therapeutics." In *The Social Basis of Health and Healing in Africa*, ed. S. Feierman and J. M. Janzen, 339–365. Berkeley: University of California Press.

Probst, Peter. 1999. "*Mchape* '95, or, The Sudden Fame of Billy Goodson Chisupe: Healing, Social Memory and the Enigma of the Public Sphere in Post-Banda Malawi." *Africa* 69 (1): 108–138.

Purcell, Trevor, and Elizabeth Akinyi Onjoro. 2002. "Indigenous Knowledge, Power and Parity: Models of Knowledge Integration." In *Participating in Development: Approaches to Indigenous Knowledge*, ed. P. Sillitoe, A. Bicker, and J. Pottier, 162–188. London: Routledge.

Ramsay, F. Jeffress. 2004. *Global Studies: Africa*. 10th ed. Guilford, Conn.: McGraw-Hill/Dushkin.

Ranger, Terence O. 1966. "Witchcraft Eradication Movements in Central and Southern Tanzania and Their Connection with the Maji Maji Rising." Seminar Paper, University College, Dar es Salaam.

———. 1967. *Revolt in Southern Rhodesia, 1896–7: A Study in African Resistance*. London: Heinemann.

———. 1983. "The Invention of Tradition in Colonial Africa." In *The Invention of Tra-*

dition, ed. E. J. Hobsbawm and T. O. Ranger, 211–262. Cambridge: Cambridge University Press.

——. 1986. "Religious Movements and Politics in Sub-Saharan Africa." *African Studies Review* 29 (2): 1–69.

——. 1993. "The Invention of Tradition Revisited: The Case of Colonial Africa." In *Legitimacy and the State in Twentieth-Century Africa,* ed. Terence Ranger and Olufeni Vaughan, 62–111. London: Macmillan.

Rasmussen, Susan J. 1998. "Only Women Know the Trees: Medicine Women and the Role of Herbal Healing in Tuareg Culture." *Journal of Anthropological Research* 54 (2): 147–171.

——. 2001a. *Healing in Community.* Westport, Conn.: Bergin & Garvey.

——. 2001b. "Betrayal or Affirmation? Transformations in Witchcraft Technologies of Power, Danger and Agency among the Tuareg of Niger." In *Magical Interpretations, Material Realities: Modernity, Witchcraft, and the Occult in Postcolonial Africa,* ed. H. L. Moore and T. Sanders, 136–159. New York: Routledge.

Redmayne, Alison. 1970. "Chikanga: An African Diviner with an International Reputation." In *Witchcraft Confessions & Accusations,* ed. M. Douglas, 103–128. London and New York: Tavistock Publications.

Reis, Ria. 2000. "The 'Wounded Healer' as Ideology: The Work of Ngoma in Swaziland." In *The Quest for Fruition through Ngoma: The Political Aspects of Healing in Southern Africa,* ed. R. van Dijk, R. Reis, and M. Spierenburg, 61–75. Athens: Ohio University Press.

Rekdal, Ole Bjørn. 1999. "Cross-Cultural Healing in East African Ethnography." *Medical Anthropology Quarterly* 13 (4): 458–482.

Reynolds, Pamela. 1986. "The Training of Traditional Healers in Mashonaland." In *The Professionalisation of African Medicine,* ed. M. Last and G. L. Chavunduka, 165–187. Manchester and Dover, N.H.: Manchester University Press in association with the International African Institute.

——. 1996. *Traditional Healers and Childhood in Zimbabwe.* Athens, Ohio: Ohio University Press.

Richards, Audrey. 1935/1970. "A Modern Movement of Witch-Finders." In *Witchcraft and Sorcery,* ed. M. G. Marwick, 201–212. Harmondsworth: Penguin.

Ridder, Trudy de. 1997. "The Trauma of Testifying: Deponent's Difficult Healing Process." *Track Two* 6 (3–4): 30–33.

Roseman, Marina. 1988. "The Pragmatics of Aesthetics." *Social Science and Medicine* 27 (8): 811–818.

——. 1991. *Healing Sounds from the Malaysian Rainforest: Temiar Music and Medicine.* Berkeley: University of California Press.

Ross, Fiona. 2003. *Bearing Witness: Women and the Truth and Reconciliation Commission.* London: Pluto Press.

Rudolph, S. H., and J. Piscatori, eds. 1997. *Transnational Religion and Fading States.* Boulder, Colo.: Westview Press.

Sanders, Todd. 2001. "Save Our Skins: Structural Adjustment, Morality and the Occult in Tanzania." In *Magical Interpretations, Material Realities: Modernity, Witchcraft and the Occult in Postcolonial Africa,* ed. H. L. Moore and T. Sanders, 160–183. New York: Routledge.

Scarnecchia, Timothy. 1997. "Mai Chaza's Guta re Jehova (City of God)." *Journal of Southern African Studies* 23 (1): 87–105.

Scarry, Elaine. 1985. *The Body in Pain: The Making and Unmaking of the World.* New York: Oxford University Press.

Schapera, I. 1953. "Some Comments on Comparative Method in Anthropology." *American Anthropologist* 55 (3): 353–362.

Schoenbrun, David Lee. 1997. *The Historical Reconstruction of Great Lakes Bantu Cultural Vocabulary: Etymologies and Reconstructions.* Sprache und Geschichte in Afrika, Beiheft 9. Cologne: Ruediger Koeppe Verlag.

———. 1998. *A Green Place, a Good Place: Agrarian Change, Gender, and Social Identity in the Great Lakes Region to the 15th Century.* Portsmouth, N.H.: Heinemann.

———. 2001. "Comment on Ehret, 'Bantu Expansions.'" *The International Journal of African Historical Studies* 34 (1): 56–61.

Schoepf, Brooke G. 2001. "International AIDS Research in Anthropology: Taking a Critical Perspective on the Crisis." *Annual Review of Anthropology* 30 (1): 335–361.

Schoffeleers, Matthew. 1991. "Ritual Healing and Political Acquiescence: The Case of the Zionist Churches in Southern Africa." *Africa* 60 (1): 1–25.

———. 1992. *River of Blood: The Genesis of a Martyr Cult in Southern Malawi, c. AD 1600.* Madison: University of Wisconsin Press.

———. 1994. "Christ in African Folk Theology: The Nganga Paradigm." In *Religion in Africa: Experience and Expression,* ed. Thomas D. Blakely, Walter E. A. van Beek, and Dennis L. Thomson, 73–88. London and Portsmouth, N.H.: James Currey and Heinemann.

Schumaker, Lyn. 2001. *Africanizing Anthropology: Fieldwork, Networks, and the Making of Cultural Knowledge in Central Africa.* Durham, N.C.: Duke University Press.

Selolwane, O. 1998. "Equality of Citizenship and the Gendering of Democracy in Botswana." In *Botswana: Politics and Society,* ed. W. A. Edge and M. H. Lekorwe. Pretoria: J. L. van Schaik Publishers.

———. 2001. "From Infrastructural Development to Privatization: Employment Creation and Poverty Reduction in Gaborone." Paper presented at the ASC Conference on African Urban Economies, Leiden, the Netherlands, November 9–11, 2001.

Semali, I. A. J. 1986. "Associations and Healers: Attitudes towards Collaboration in Tanzania." In *The Professionalisation of African Medicine,* ed. M. Last and G. L. Chavunduka, 87–97. Manchester: International African Institute.

Setel, Philip. 1999. *A Plague of Paradoxes: AIDS, Culture, and Demography in Northern Tanzania.* Chicago: University of Chicago Press.

Shapin, Steven, and Simon Schaffer. 1985. *Leviathan and the Air-Pump: Hobbes, Boyle, and the Experimental Life.* Princeton, N.J.: Princeton University Press.

Sharp, Lesley Alexandra. 1993. *The Possessed and the Dispossessed: Spirits, Identity, and Power in a Madagascar Migrant Town.* Berkeley: University of California Press.

Shaw, Rosalind. 2002. *Memories of the Slave Trade: Ritual and the Historical Imagination in Sierra Leone.* Chicago: University of Chicago Press.

Shaw, Rosalind, and Charles Stewart. 1994. "Introduction: Problematizing Syncretism." In *Syncretism/Anti-syncretism: The Politics of Religious Synthesis,* ed. C. Stewart and R. Shaw, 1–26. London and New York: Routledge.

Shay, Donald. 1995. *Achilles in Vietnam: Combat Trauma and the Undoing of Character.* New York: Scribner.

Sillitoe, Paul. 1998. "The Development of Indigenous Knowledge." *Current Anthropology* 39 (2): 223–252.

Silva, Calane da. 1975. "Liquidar o Obscurantismo mas Aproveitar o que Há de Positivo." *Tempo* 229 (16 February).

Simon, Chris, and Masilo Lamla. 1991. "Merging Pharmacopoeia." *Journal of Ethnopharmacology* 33 (3): 237–242.

Skinner, Donald. 1998. *Apartheid's Violent Legacy: A Report on Trauma in the Western Cape.* Cape Town, South Africa: Trauma Centre for Victims of Violence and Torture.

Smith, Wilfred Cantwell. 1977. *Belief and History.* Charlottesville: University Press of Virginia.

Somé, Malidoma Patrice. 1998. *The Healing Wisdom of Africa.* New York: J. P. Tarcher.

Sousa, José Augusto Alves de. 1991. *Os Jesuítas em Moçambique, 1541–1991: No Quintenário do Quarto Período da Nossa Missão.* Braga: Livraria Apostolado da Imprensa.

Spierenburg, M. 2001. "Moving into Another Spirit Province: Immigrants and the Mhondoro Cult in Northern Zimbabwe." In *Mobile Africa: Changing Patterns of Movement in Africa and Beyond,* ed. M. de Bruijn, R. van Dijk, and D. Foeken. Leiden: Brill.

Stephen, Michele. 1996. "The Mekeo 'Man of Sorrow': Sorcery and the Individuation of the Self." *American Ethnologist* 23 (1): 83–101.

Stirling, Leader. 1947. *Bush Doctor: Universities' Mission to Central Africa.* London: Parrett and Neves.

———. 1977. *Tanzanian Doctor.* London and Nairobi: Heinemann.

Stirrat, R. L. 1998. "Response to Paul Sillitoe's 'The Development of Indigenous Knowledge: A New Applied Anthropology'." *Current Anthropology* 39 (2): 242–243.

Stoller, Paul. 1989. *Fusion of the Worlds: An Ethnography of Possession among the Songhay of Niger.* Chicago: University of Chicago Press.

———. 1996. "Sounds and Things: Pulsations of Power in Songhay." In *The Performance of Healing,* ed. C. Laderman and M. Roseman, 165–184. New York: Routledge.

Stone, Martin. 1985. "Shellshock and the Psychologists." In *The Anatomy of Madness: Essays in the History of Psychiatry,* vol. 2, ed. W. F. Bynum, Roy Porter, and Michael Shepherd. London and New York: Tavistock.

Summerfield, Derek. 1999. "A Critique of Seven Assumptions behind Psychological Trauma Programmes in War-Affected Areas." *Social Science & Medicine* 48 (10): 1449–1462.

Sundkler, Bengt G. M. 1961. *Bantu Prophets in South Africa.* 2nd ed. London: Oxford University Press.

———. 1976. *Zulu Zion and Some Swazi Zionists.* London: Oxford University Press.

Swantz, Marja-Liisa. 1989. "Manipulation of Multiple Health Systems in the Coastal Regions of Tanzania." In *Culture, Experience, and Pluralism: Essays on African Ideas of Illness and Healing,* ed. A. Jacobson-Widding and D. Westerlund, 277–288. Uppsala: Academiae Upsaliensis.

Swartz, Leslie, Gibson Kerry, and Rob Sandenbergh. 2002. *Counselling and Coping.* Oxford: Oxford University Press.

Taussig, Michael. 1992. *The Nervous System.* London: Routledge.

Thomas, Linda E. 1994. "African Indigenous Churches as a Source of Socio-Political Transformation in South Africa." *Africa Today* 41 (1): 39–56.

Toit, Brian du. 1998. "Modern Folk Medicine in South Africa." *South African Journal of Ethnology* 21 (4): 145–152.

Truth and Reconciliation Commission. 1996a. *Interim Report of the Truth and Reconciliation Commission.* Cape Town, South Africa: TRC.

———. 1996b. *Policy Framework for Urgent Interim Reparation Measures.* Cape Town, South Africa: TRC.

Turner, Victor. 1967. *The Forest of Symbols: Aspects of Ndembu Ritual.* Ithaca, N.Y.: Cornell University Press.

———. 1968. *The Drums of Affliction: A Study of Religious Processes among the Ndembu of Zambia.* Oxford: Clarendon.

Ulluwishewa, Rohana. 1993. "Indigenous Knowledge, National IK Resource Centres and Sustainable Development." *Indigenous Knowledge & Development Monitor* 1 (3): 11–13.

Ulmera, L., L. Ramirez, Y. Lafort, F. Machobo, J. Pfeiffer, and S. Gloyd. 1994. "Manica Province Child Nutrition Survey." Chimoio, Mozambique: Mozambique Mental Health Committee and Manica Provincial Health Directorate.

UNDP (United Nations Development Programme). *Human Development Report 1995: Gender and Human Development.* New York: Oxford University Press, 1995.

UNICEF. 1994. *Children and Women in Zimbabwe: A Situation Analysis.* Harare, Zimbabwe: UNICEF.

Veer, Peter van der, ed. 1996. *Conversion to Modernities: The Globalization of Christianity.* New York: Routledge.

Vansina, Jan. 1990. *Paths in the Rainforests.* Madison: University of Wisconsin Press.

———. 2001. "Comment on Ehret, 'Bantu Expansions.'" *The International Journal of African Historical Studies* 34 (1): 52–54.

Vaughan, Megan. 1991. *Curing Their Ills: Colonial Power and African Illness.* Stanford, Calif.: Stanford University Press.

Vertovec, S. 2001. "Transnationalism and Identity." *Journal of Ethnic and Migration Studies* 27 (4): 573–582.

Vines, Alex. 1991. *RENAMO: Terrorism in Mozambique.* London: James Currey.

Vines, Alex, and K. Wilson. 1995. "Churches and the Peace Process in Mozambique." In *The Christian Churches and the Democratization of Africa,* ed. Paul Gifford. Leiden: E. J. Brill.

Von Doepp, P. 1998. "The Kingdom Beyond Zasintha: Churches and Political Life in Malawi's Post-Authoritarian Era." In *Democratization in Malawi: A Stocktaking,* ed. K. M. Phiri and H. K. R. Ross. Blantyre: Christian Literature Association in Malawi.

Wafer, James William. 1991. *The Taste of Blood: Spirit Possession in Brazilian Candomblé.* Philadelphia: University of Pennsylvania Press.

Waite, Gloria. 2000. "Traditional Medicine and the Quest for National Identity in Zimbabwe." *Zambezia* 27 (2): 235–268.

Walshe, Peter. 1991. "South Africa: Prophetic Christianity and the Liberation Movement." *The Journal of Modern African Studies* 29 (1): 27–60.

Werbner, Richard. 1989. *Ritual Passage, Sacred Journey: The Process and Organization of Religious Movement.* Washington, D.C.: Smithsonian Institution Press.

———. 2002a. "Citizenship and the Politics of Recognition in Botswana." In *Minorities in the Millennium: Perspectives from Botswana,* ed. I. N. Mazonde. Gaborone, Botswana: Lightbooks.

———. 2002b. "Challenging Minorities: Difference and Tribal Citizenship in Botswana." *Journal of Southern African Studies* 28 (4): 671–684.

Werbner, Richard, ed. 1977. *Regional Cults.* Association of Social Anthropologists of the Commonwealth Monograph 16. London: Academic Press.

———. 1998. *Memory and the Postcolony: African Anthropology and the Critique of Power.* London: Zed Books.

West, Harry G. 2005. *Kupilikula: Governance and the Invisible Realm in Mozambique.* Chicago: University of Chicago Press.

White, Luise. 1994. "Blood Brotherhood Revisited: Kinship, Relationship, and the Body in East and Central Africa." *Africa* 64 (3): 359–372.

———. 1995. " 'They Could Make their Victims Dull': Genders and Genres, Fantasies and Cures in Colonial Southern Uganda." *American Historical Review* 100 (5): 1379–1402.

———. 1997. "The Traffic in Heads: Bodies, Borders and the Articulation of Regional Histories." *Journal of Southern African Studies* 23 (2): 325–338.

———. 2000. *Speaking with Vampires: Rumor and History in Colonial Africa.* Berkeley, Calif.: University of California Press.

Whyte, Susan Reynolds. 1982. "Penicillin, Battery Acid and Sacrifice: Cures and Causes in Nyole Medicine." *Social Science and Medicine* 16: 2055–2064.

———. 1988. "The Power of Medicines in East Africa." In *The Context of Medicines in Developing Countries: Studies in Pharmaceutical Anthropology,* ed. S. van der Geest and S. R. Whyte, 217–233. Dordrecht: Kluwer Academic Publishers.

———. 1997. *Questioning Misfortune: The Pragmatics of Uncertainty in Eastern Uganda.* Cambridge: Cambridge University Press.

Whyte, Susan Reynolds, and Harriet Birungi. 2000. "The Business of Medicines and the Politics of Knowledge in Uganda." In *Global Health Policy, Local Realities: The Fallacy of the Level Playing Field,* ed. Linda Whiteford and Lenore Manderson. Boulder, Colo.: Lynne Reinner.

Whyte, Susan Reynolds, and Sjaak van der Geest. 1988. "Medicines in Context: An Introduction." In *The Context of Medicines in Developing Countries: Studies in Pharmaceutical Anthropology,* ed. S. van der Geest and S. R. Whyte, 3–11. Dordrecht: Kluwer Academic Publishers.

Whyte, Susan Reynolds, Sjaak van der Geest, and Anita Hardon. 2002. *Social Lives of Medicines.* Cambridge: Cambridge University Press.

Willis, Roy G. 1968. "Kamcape: An Anti-Sorcery Movement in South-west Tanzania." *Africa* 38 (1): 1–15.

Willis, Roy G., and K. B. S. Chisanga. 1999. *Some Spirits Heal, Others Only Dance: A Journey into Human Selfhood in an African Village.* Oxford and New York: Berg.

Wilson, Richard. 2001. *The Politics of Truth and Reconciliation in South Africa: Legitimizing the Post-Apartheid State.* Cambridge: Cambridge University Press.

Wolf, Eric. 1982. *Europe and the People without History.* Berkeley: University of California Press.

World Bank. 2001. *World Development Report 2000–2001: Attacking Poverty.* Oxford: Oxford University Press.

World Health Organization. 1978. *The Promotion and Development of Traditional Medicine: Report of a WHO Meeting.* Geneva: World Health Organization.

———. 1989. *Report of a WHO Informal Consultation on Traditional Medicine and AIDS: In Vitro Screening for Anti-HIV Activity.* Geneva: World Health Organization.

———. 1995. *Traditional Practitioners as Primary Health Care Workers.* Geneva: World Health Organization.

Yamba, C. Bawa. 1997. "Cosmologies in Turmoil: Witchfinding and AIDS in Chiawa, Zambia." *Africa* 67 (2): 200.

Young, Allan. 1995. *Harmony of Illusions: Inventing Post-Traumatic Stress Disorder.* Princeton, N.J.: Princeton University Press.

Contributors

Christopher J. Colvin is a postdoctoral fellow at the Center for Comparative Literature and Society at Columbia University. His current research interests include apartheid reparations, psychological discourses of trauma, and images and narratives of suffering.

Rijk van Dijk is an anthropologist working at the African Studies Centre, Leiden. He is author of *Young Malawian Puritans* and co-editor of *The Quest for Fruition through Ngoma; Mobile Africa;* and *Situating Globality: African Agency in the Appropriation of Global Culture.*

Steven Feierman is Professor of History and Sociology of Science and Professor of History at the University of Pennsylvania. He is author of *Peasant Intellectuals* and *The Shambaa Kingdom*, co-editor of *The Social Basis of Health and Healing in Africa,* and co-author of *African History: From Earliest Times to Independence.*

Stacey Langwick is Assistant Professor of Anthropology and Women's Studies and Gender Research at the University of Florida. Her current research examines the political, economic, social, and technical factors that have shaped medical pluralism in contemporary Tanzania.

Tracy J. Luedke is Assistant Professor of Anthropology at Northeastern Illinois University. Her research addresses the ways individual and social bodies figure in Christianized healing in Mozambique.

Julian M. Murchison is Assistant Professor of Anthropology and Sociology at Millsaps College. His research interests include the role of religious and moral imaginations in understandings and experiences of health and illness.

James Pfeiffer is Associate Professor in the Department of Health Services at the University of Washington's School of Public Health and Community Medicine. He also works with Health Alliance International as Director of Mozambique Operations in their efforts to support AIDS treatment expansion in Mozambique's national scale-up plan.

David Simmons is Assistant Professor of Anthropology and Public Health at the University of South Carolina, Columbia. As a specialist in the study of health inequities, he has also been involved in projects or research on HIV/

AIDS, maternal and child health, water and sanitation, and health and human rights.

Harry G. West is Lecturer in Anthropology at the School of Oriental and African Studies, University of London. He is co-editor of *Transparency and Conspiracy: Ethnographies of Suspicion in the New World Order* and author of *Kupilikula: Governance and the Invisible Realm in Mozambique.*

Index

bique, traditional healing and Pentecostal and African Independent Churches (AICs) in
Piscatori, J., 103
Plotkin, Mark J., 40n4
Poewe, Karla, 104
post-traumatic stress disorder (PTSD), 176
Probst, Peter, 129–30
professionalism and traditional medicine, 68–69, 75, 76–77, 78

Ranger, Terence O., 17n5, 165n17, 192
Rekdal, Ole Bjørn, 19n15
RENAMO (Resistência Nacional Moçambicana), 21–22, 43, 55, 59
Richards, Audrey, 4
Rudolph, S. H., 103

Sanders, Todd, 84, 100n3, 120
Scarnecchia, Timothy, 18n9
Scarry, Elaine, 63n1
Schapera, Isaac, 186
Schoepf, Brooke G., 138
Schoffeleers, Matthew, 192
Shaw, Rosalind, 18n13
Shembe, Isaiah, 189
Sillitoe, Paul, 37
Simon, Chris, 19n21
Sitimi, Enoch, 109
Smith, Wilfred Cantwell, 37
sorcery. See witchcraft
South Africa and traumatic storytelling, 166–84; the Cape Town Trauma Centre, 171–75, 176–80, 181–82; criminal violence and traumatic storytelling, 176, 182; defining traumatic storytelling, 168–69; global spread of traumatic storytelling, 168; *i-nevs* (nerves) and trauma, 174; institutional agendas and traumatic storytelling, 181–82; intractability of traumatic storytelling, 180–81; the Khulumani Support Group, 172–73, 174–75, 176–80, 182–83; and the medical language of trauma, 179–80; nerves and witchcraft, 174–75; the political economy of traumatic storytelling, 167–69, 181; and post-traumatic stress disorder, 176; post-TRC projects and storytelling strategies, 171–73; the reparations issue, 179–80; rural outreach and trauma-related services, 176–78; split between the Trauma Centre and Khulumani, 178–80, 182; therapeutic vocabularies, 174–75; trauma discourse in the townships and public health facilities, 174, 175–76; and trauma theory, 167–68;

the TRC, 166, 167–68, 169–71, 181; the TRC and international networks, 169–70; the TRC and mental health community/therapeutic ethic, 170, 184n6; the TRC and "right of recountability," 168, 183n4; the TRC and victim hearings, 170–71; the TRC as medico-political art form, 169–71
South Africa's Truth and Reconciliation Commission (TRC), 166, 167–68, 169–71, 181, 183n1. *See also* South Africa and traumatic storytelling
Speaking with Vampires (White), 130–31
Stamps, Timothy, 75
Stewart, Charles, 18n13
Stirling, Leader. *See* Tanganyika, colonial, and the boundary between traditional medicine and biomedicine

TAMOFA (The Tanzania Mozambique Friendship Association), 29
Tanganyika, colonial, and the boundary between traditional medicine and biomedicine, 143–65; botanicals and herbal medicines, 160–62; building projects and Stirling's expansion of biomedicine, 150–55; the contours of traditional medicine, 159–63; porousness of boundaries separating biomedicine and traditional medicine, 144, 155–59; and problems of authority in colonial Tanganyika, 144, 164n5; purification and mediation, 157–59; Stirling's accounts and scientific knowledge/assertion of biomedicine, 145–46; Stirling's depictions of initiation ceremonies, 149–50; Stirling's life and books, 145–46, 164nn6,7; Stirling's representations of nature, 146–49; witchcraft and witchcraft eradication movements, 158–59, 165n17
Tanganyikan African National Union (TANU), 145
Tanzanian Doctor (Stirling), 145, 146–48, 149, 151, 153, 155, 156, 160, 162
Tanzanian narratives about HIV/AIDS, 125–42; biomedicine and traditional healing, 132–34, 142n10; and epilepsy, 140; and fertility problems, 139–40; and the figure of the Western doctor (Dr. Ansgar), 132–34, 135–36, 137; HIV testing, 133, 135–36; and linguistic boundaries (Kingoni and Kiswahili languages), 135, 142n11; and the local landscape of "modern" Peramiho and the village of Mgazini, 134; Mama Asante's stories of *dawa ya ukimwi* (AIDS medicine/